BACKYARD
PHARMACY

Inspiring | Educating | Creating | Entertaining

Brimming with creative inspiration, how-to projects, and useful
information to enrich your everyday life, Quarto Knows is a favorite
destination for those pursuing their interests and passions. Visit our
site and dig deeper with our books into your area of interest:
Quarto Creates, Quarto Cooks, Quarto Homes, Quarto Lives,
Quarto Drives, Quarto Explores, Quarto Gifts, or Quarto Kids.

Acquisitions Editor: Billie Brownell

Senior Art Director: Brad Springer

Layout: Diana Boger

Front Cover Design: Laura Drew

Cover photo: Anita Oberhauser;
     Getty Images

First published in 2015 by Cool Springs Press, an imprint of The Quarto Group, 401
Second Avenue North, Suite 310, Minneapolis, MN 55401 USA. T (612) 344-8100
F (612) 344-8692 www.QuartoKnows.com

Cool Springs Press titles are also available at discount for retail, wholesale,
promotional, and bulk purchase. For details, contact the Special Sales Manager by
email at specialsales@quarto.com or by mail at The Quarto Group, Attn: Special Sales
Manager, 401 Second Avenue North, Suite 310, Minneapolis, MN 55401 USA.

This book provides general information on various widely known and widely
accepted home remedies. However, it should not be relied upon as recommending or
promoting any specific diagnosis or method of treatment for a particular condition,
and it is not intended as a substitute for medical advice or for direct diagnosis
and treatment of a medical condition by a qualified physician. Readers who have
questions about a particular condition, possible treatments for that condition, or
possible reactions from the condition or from any treatment for the condition should
consult a physician or other qualified healthcare professional. In addition, since
reactions to the ingredients in the home remedies described in this book may vary
from person to person, it is the reader's responsibility to check the ingredients for a
home remedy prior to use to determine if any ingredient may cause any allergic or
other adverse reaction.

Except for the publisher's website associated with this work, the publisher is not
affiliated with and does not sponsor or endorse any websites, organizations or
other sources of information referred to herein, and the publisher and the authors
do not warrant the accuracy, completeness or currency of any information or
recommendations provided by those sources.

The authors and the publisher shall not be liable for any damages allegedly arising
from the information in this book, and they specifically disclaim any liability from
the use or application of any of the contents of this book.

Library of Congress Cataloging-in-Publication Data

Millard, Elizabeth, author.
  Backyard pharmacy : growing medicinal plants in your own yard / Elizabeth Millard.
    pages cm
  Other title: Growing medicinal plants in your own yard
  Includes index.
  ISBN 978-1-59186-596-4 (sc)
  1. Medicinal plants. 2. Gardening. I. Title. II. Title: Growing medicinal plants in
your own yard.

SB293.M55 2015
633.8'8--dc23

ISBN: 978-1-59186-596-4

2014044870

Printed in USA

BACKYARD PHARMACY

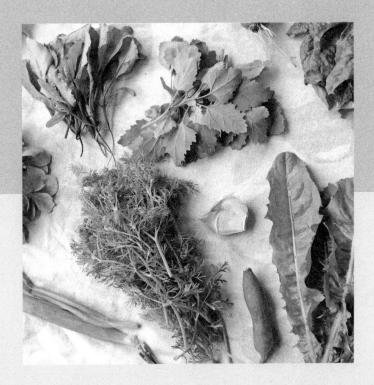

Growing Medicinal Plants in Your Own Yard

ELIZABETH MILLARD

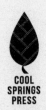

COOL SPRINGS PRESS

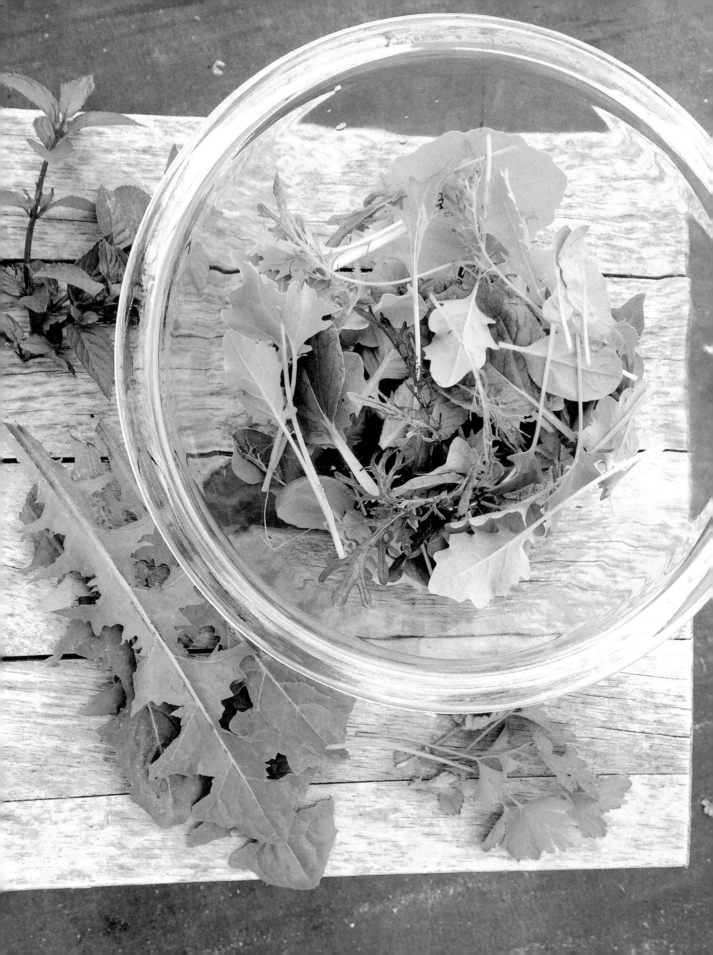

For Bossy K,
always

This book was written in the middle of farming season while my fantastic partner, Karla Pankow, and I were living in a camper on rented land with our two dogs, Idgy and Ruthie. It took an inordinate amount of patience and fortitude—and I don't mean on my part. So, thanks first of all to the best Bossy of all, and our very supportive pups.

Thanks, too, to my editor Billie Brownell, and to Cool Springs Press, for shepherding this project out the camper door.

Also, I owe a deep level of gratitude to the thousands—even millions—of growers who came before me and were such artful stewards of the land. Farmers, foragers, herbalists, gardeners, and healers, I thank you all.

Contents

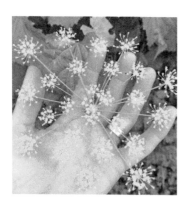

1. The Basics of Gardening . 11

2. Using Your Harvest . 33

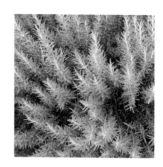

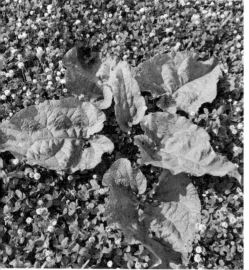

3. Kitchen Garden Herbs . 45

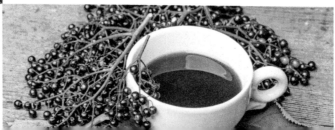

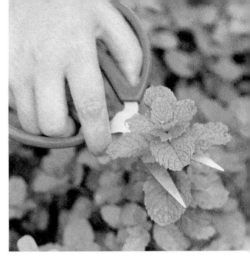

4. Herbal Garden Remedies . 87

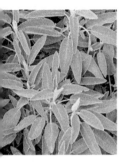

5. Fruits and Shrubs . 133

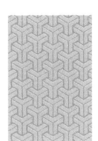

6. Wild Yard Friends . 155

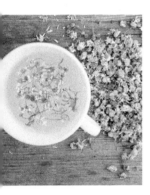

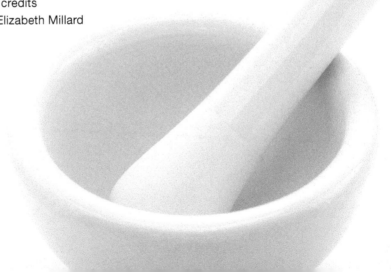

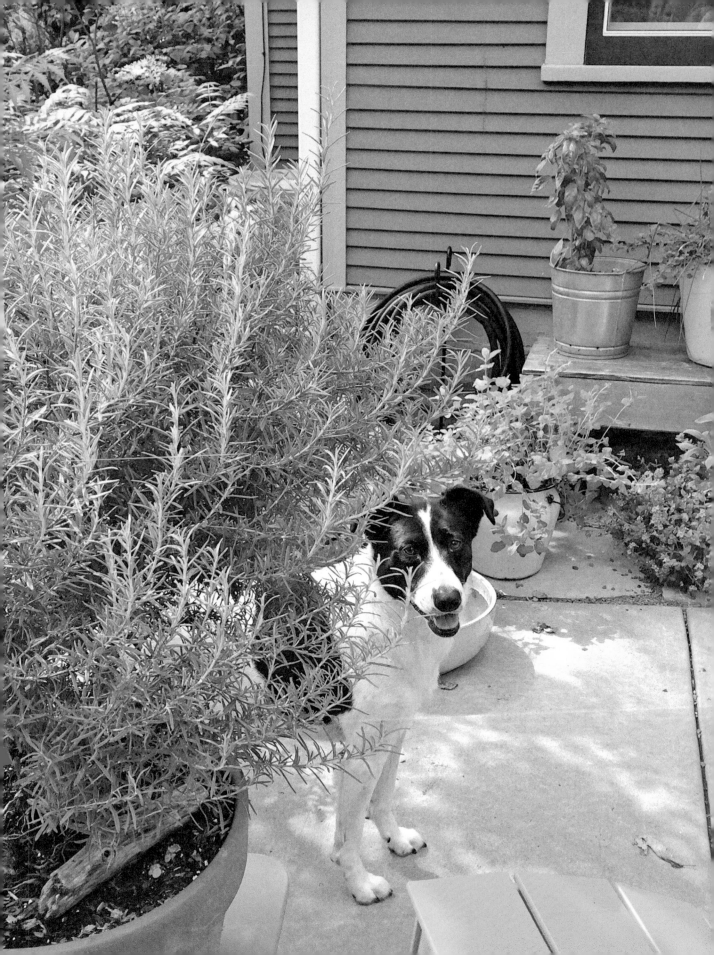

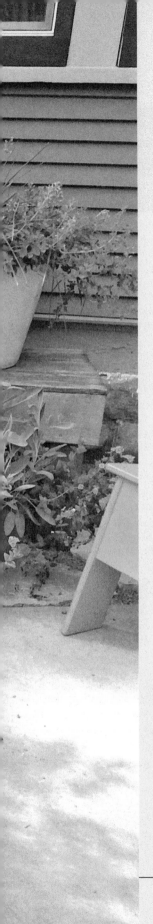

Introduction

My adventure with medicinal plants began with a very simple preparation of dandelion leaves, red clover, and plantain, roughly shredded and mashed together with some apple juice, and left to ferment in the sun for a few hours. I was in kindergarten. The potion was supposed to help my friend Val win the love of her unrequited crush, Bruce, and when I got stung by a bee while picking the clover, I took it as a sign that this would be a powerful brew indeed. Unfortunately, he refused to drink it, trashing my reputation as a budding herbalist. Thanks for nothing, Bruce.

Since then, I've used herbs and other medicinal plants for more realistic purposes like soothing sore muscles, improving digestion, banishing headaches, and addressing the approximately one million mosquito bites I get every summer at Bossy Acres, the farm I own with my partner, Karla Pankow. Every year, we experiment with new varieties of medicinal plants like valerian, calendula, chamomile, and yarrow growing alongside culinary favorites like basil and thyme.

Although I'm not a professional herbalist—yet—I've been fond of herbs since that first failed potion, and our little medicinal garden at Bossy Acres feels like a revelation every growing season. For meals, we throw a collection of plants together that includes both cultivated and wild selections, so lambs quarters might cozy up to peppermint, with grilled garlic bringing it all together. It's not uncommon for guests to start a dinner discussion with, "Now, *what* am I eating?"

In addition to being useful, medicinal plants can also make an outdoor living space look more vibrant.

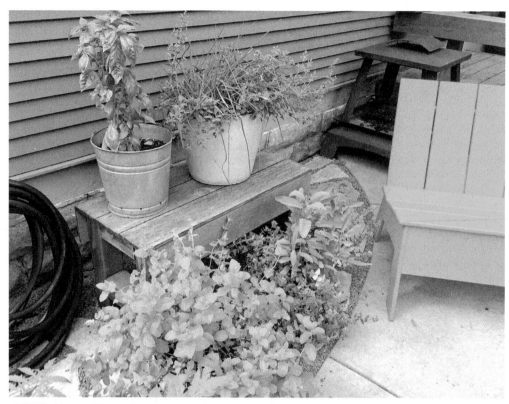

Three small bundles of thyme, ready to give as gifts, or for use in a preparation.

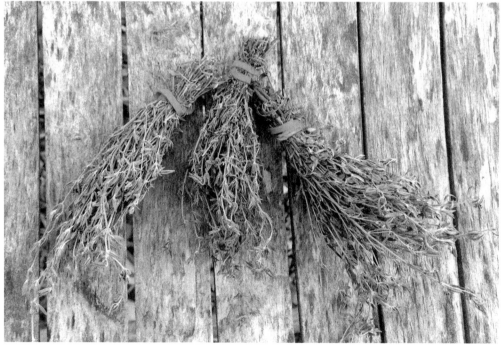

Part of the appeal of medicinals for me comes from being drawn to self-sufficiency, sustainability, and better control over my health. I've always been an advocate of health-care over sick-care, and part of that difference springs from preventative measures—staying de-stressed, connecting with nature, sleeping well, eating real food, and using plants with known medicinal properties for boosting immunity and reducing inflammation. To me, all of these strategies are interconnected.

I'm also humbled to be connected to a deep, rich history of medicinal tradition. For centuries, plants have been used in ritual and healing. Some of the oldest documents from Chinese and Egyptian culture describe medicinal uses of plants, and recently the World Health Organization estimated that 80 percent of people worldwide still rely on herbal medicines for some aspect of their health care.

In terms of my own medicinal uses, you'll find that I'm particularly fond of very simple remedies. I greatly admire herbalists who create five-herb blends that address specific conditions, but I gravitate toward one-herb, one-purpose kind of uses. If I have a sore throat, I gargle with a mix of hot water and crushed, dried cayenne. For those mosquito bites, I chew a plantain leaf and put the mushy result on them. I've tried to create more combinations, but always find myself drifting back to easier approaches, usually resulting in lots and lots of tea.

As a gardener and farmer, I take the same strategy as I do with medicinal preparations: if it's easy to grow, it wins my love. At Bossy Acres, we grow about sixty different

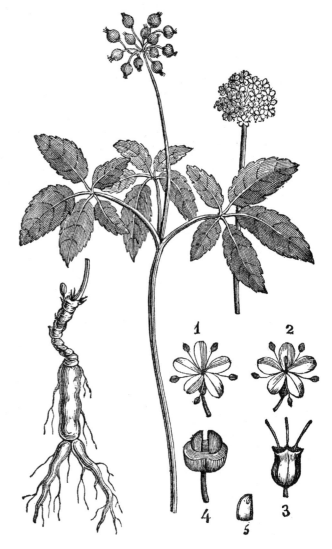

vegetables, some fruits, and around twenty to thirty herbs per year, so any plant that needs a wealth of attention tends to get knocked out of the lineup.

For this book, I chose my favorite plants based on ease of growing, medicinal efficacy, one-herb remedies, and personal fondness. Rather than focus exclusively on herbs, I've included some other major plants that have plenty of medicinal uses. Berry bushes, for example, are often overlooked when it comes to wellness, but because of their longevity and whole-plant usefulness, it's great to include them in a backyard plan.

Each chapter covers plant history, simple preparations, planting and growing considerations, and storage tips. Enjoy your herbal adventures, and if you discover a love potion in the process, definitely let me know.

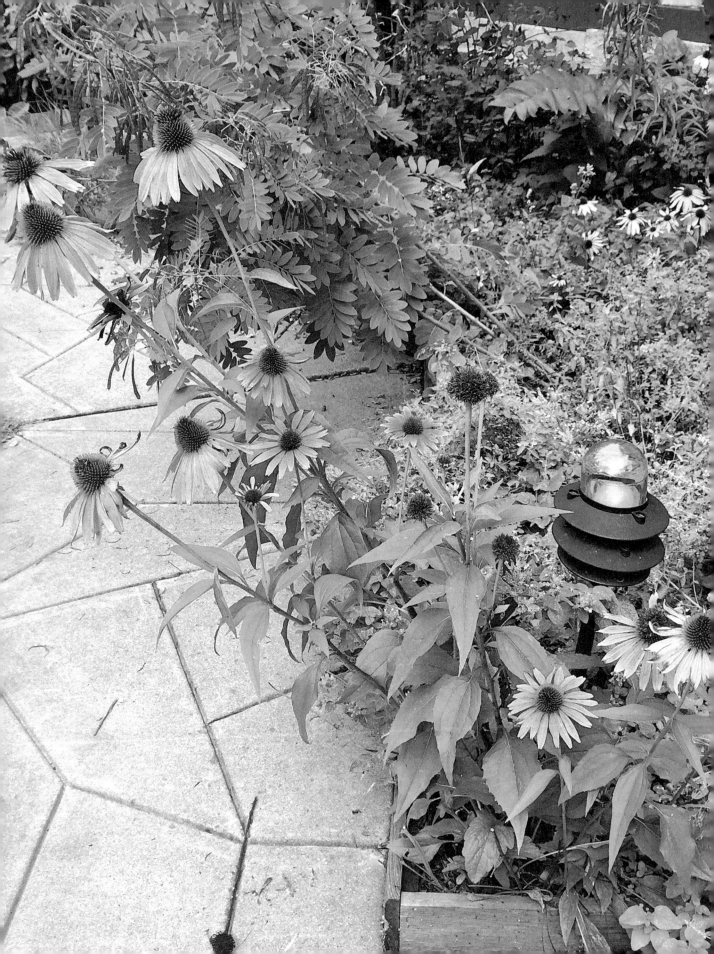

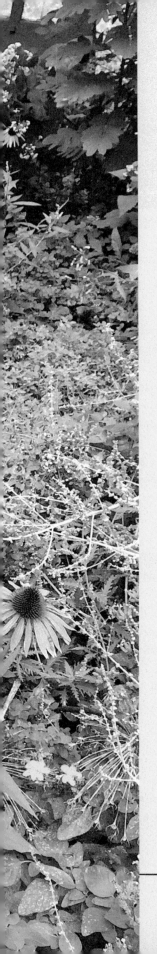

ONE

The Basics of Gardening

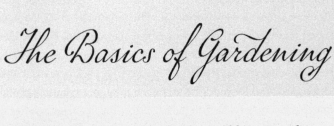

We grow an array of robust vegetables on our farm that take up plenty of space, like the pumpkins that send out thick runner stems, or the alien-looking kohlrabi, with their heavy globes snugged into the ground.

By comparison, the section we have allocated for medicinal plants seems like a little fairy garden. The delicate fronds and cute-as-a-button flowers of chamomile wave just above the dark green, lush leaves of lemon balm, giving me plenty of ideas about how to combine the two.

The fact is that our farm could become a large-scale production enterprise (it won't) and I'd still consider this small growing space as one of the most important on the land. Perhaps it's because I harvest from this section every day, chopping a bit of oregano and basil for a dish, or grabbing a few raspberry leaves to make into a bedtime tea.Our medicinal garden has become like a friend who's always happy to see me.

People tend to grow especially fond of nurturing medicinal plants, fussing over their watering needs and soil acidity. That's not surprising, because consider the return: A backyard spot filled with wellness and culinary wonders, many of them coming back year after year, growing more sturdy and robust. Creating a garden space—even if "garden" means a windowbox of herbs in your kitchen—is distinctly soul quenching, and much less intimidating than you might think. Let's get started with some herb basics.

In smaller gardens, placing pots on wheeled bases can be handy for moving them in and out of the sun.

PERENNIAL VS. ANNUAL

Plants are either perennial or annual, with the latter meaning that they have only one life cycle per growing season, and which you need to replant the following year. This includes herbs like basil, dill, and cilantro.

Many medicinal plants are perennial, which means they can stay green all winter, especially if you bring them inside, or they go dormant after a few frosts and then come back to life in the spring. That's good news for your garden, since it means one planting of an herb can last for years. Just be sure to trim the herbs back in the fall, before the first frost, so all of the plant's energy can go into the roots and prepare for dormancy.

There's also a *biennial*, which is a plant that requires two years to complete a life cycle. This is rare in herbs, though, and I know of only two: parsley and caraway.

PLANNING

A traditional medicinal garden is often arranged according to some type of logical theme. For example, you might put culinary herbs in one section and medicinal flowers in another, or group the plants based on whether they're annual or perennial so you can till up the annual bed at the end of the season.

However you group them, just be sure to keep harvesting in mind. When I first started growing medicinals, I created a partial labyrinth that was very pretty, but had some narrow pathways in certain spots. The idea was sound—a curving wall of herbs is amazing—but by making the walkways too small, I struggled whenever trying to harvest specific plants.

Another consideration might be proximity to your house or apartment building. Most likely, you'll be harvesting from the garden plot at least a few times per week, if not every day, so putting it close to an entrance is usually best.

GROWING CONDITIONS

SUN/SHADE Many herbs and other medicinals prefer full sun, although they can tolerate shade, and there are some, like mint, that do better in shady conditions. In general, though, map out a space that gets at least six hours of sun per day.

Keep in mind that the full sun of the Midwest is certainly not like the full sun of the Pacific Northwest or the full sun of the Southwest. Most likely, you already know if your garden space could double as an oven in the summer, but if you're not sure about how much it could affect your plants, you can consider tweaking your setup to create some artificial shade options.

For example, many farmers create a "caterpillar tunnel," which means a series of simple hoops that are placed over plants, with a removable covering over that. You can drape shade cloth over the hoops on the days that are particularly hot to give the plants a break. If you only have a small section of your garden that seems to be suffering with the sun, you can even set up some large sun umbrellas in the space during the hottest parts of the day.

Most helpful, though, would be to place as many plants as possible in containers that can be moved to different parts your growing space. Even larger plants can be moved if you place the pots on wheeled carts before filling them with soil. Creating this kind of mobile garden can be very helpful for dealing with sun issues.

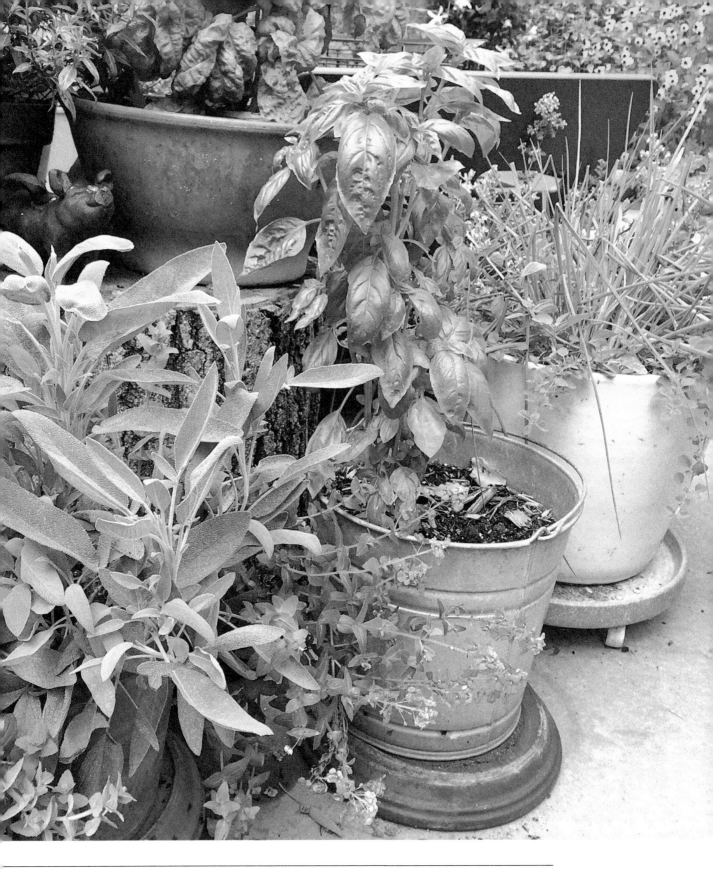

SOIL NEEDS Many medicinal plants usually prefer a moderately rich soil for growing, and appreciate well-draining soil, so if you have soil that's more like clay, or particularly dense, you may consider growing in raised beds or containers instead. If that's not an option, you can work some compost into the soil to prepare it, and add some sand or vermiculite to help with drainage. You could also try growing medicinals, such as rosemary or chamomile, in areas of your garden that have less-than-ideal soil.

If you can loosen your soil, though, it's likely you've found a good spot for your medicinal garden. Before planting, create a nutrient-rich environment by adding some fertilizer, such as fish emulsion (available at garden stores), and thoroughly mixing it into the tilled soil. Home compost is another great option, but be careful with composted manures, since these can sometimes be too high in nitrogen—herbs can grow in nitrogen-packed soil, for example, but they tend to have reduced flavor or are more susceptible to disease and pests.

To get really geeked out, test your soil's pH. This is a measure of the soil's acidity or alkalinity, and some plants have very specific requirements in terms of pH ranges. For example, thyme prefers a more alkaline environment while blueberry does better in more acidic soil.

Quick primer: on the pH range, 7.0 is considered neutral, with any measurement below that considered more acidic and above that considered more alkaline. The overall pH range is 1 to 14, and can be tested with a device that's found at any garden store (or sent to a testing lab for a more elaborate analysis).

Before planting anything in the garden, get some worm castings (worm poop), mushroom compost, or composted cow manure to rake into the soil. Spread a 1-inch layer on top of the soil and use a four-tine claw to work it in.

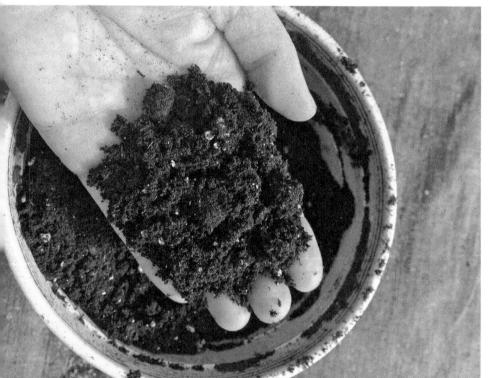

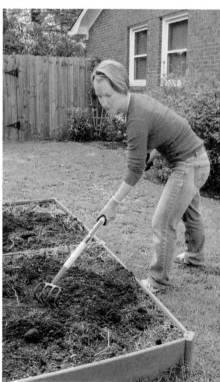

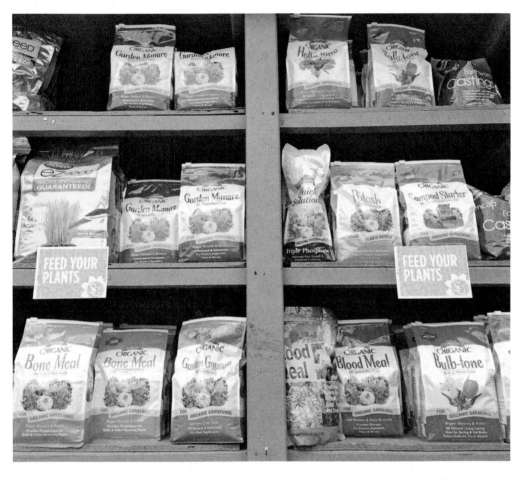

There are many options when it comes to natural fertilizers.

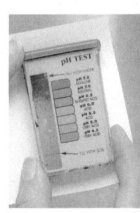

Soil test kits like this one will allow you to test your soil for pH level. Other kits will allow you to test for the presence of Nitrogen-N, Phosphorus-P, and Potassium-K in the soil.

To make the soil more alkaline, and thus increase the pH, sprinkle a little agricultural limestone (referred to as "lime") into the space and work thoroughly into the soil, or put just a touch of lime around the roots of a plant that's already established.

To increase acidity, there are many fertilizers that can be useful, such as sphagnum peat, which should be added to the topsoil around plants, or just before the planting process. You can also use what's called "elemental sulfur," but keep in mind that it's slow acting, so it may take several months to take effect. However, granular sulfur can do the trick more quickly.

If you happen to be friends with your local coffee shop owner, skip the sulfur and employ used coffee grounds instead. You'll need plenty, probably about 4 to 6 inches' worth above the soil, but it's a nice way to acidify the soil.

Maybe, at this point, your eyes are glazing over a little. I have to admit, my partner Karla is the growing nerd and loves anything involving gauges, devices, monitors, or other indicators of soil health. I'm truly more of a "plant it and see what happens" kind of girl. So, if you're more like me, then don't worry: most likely, you can plant medicinals without worrying about sweet-and-sour soil. But if your plants are struggling, soil acidity is one component worth examining.

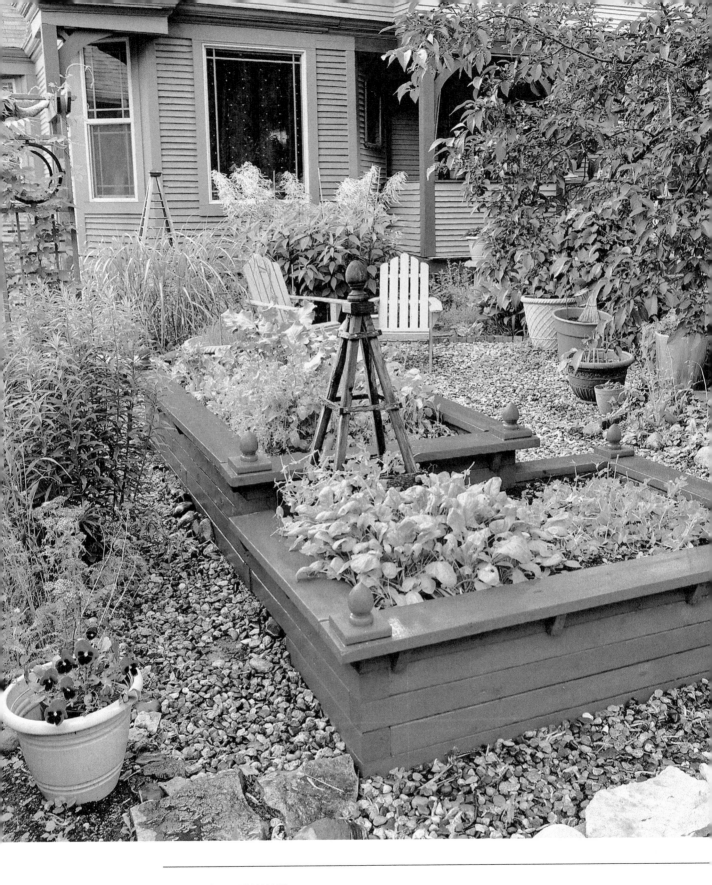

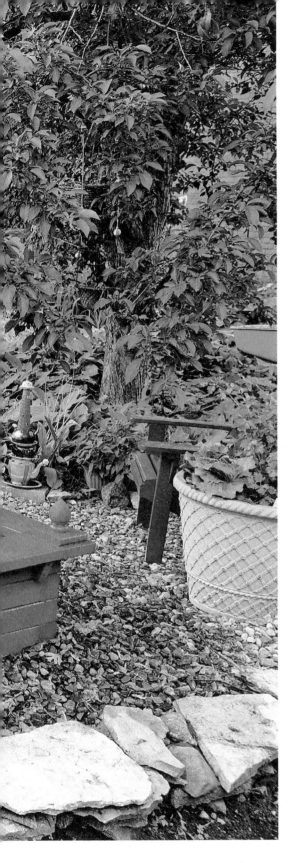

RAISED BEDS & CONTAINERS

One way to remove any doubt about your soil mix is to utilize raised beds or individual pots for your plants, flowers, and bushes. This is a perfect way to get plenty of control overwatering, drainage, fertilization, and maintenance. Also, if you're using containers, you can often bring the plants inside over the winter and extend their growing season, or you can easily reconfigure your garden space if you want to add or subtract plants.

One excellent resource if you want to go this route is *Container Gardening for All Seasons: Enjoy Year-Round Color with 101 Designs*, by Barbara Wise. Another option is my first book, *Indoor Kitchen Gardening: Turn Your Home Into a Year-Round Vegetable Garden*, which covers a number of issues when it comes to growing in pots and other containers.

Opposite: In addition to being very handy, well-designed raised beds can also become an attractive part of the garden.

Putting plants in containers can be handy when you want to move them to different parts of the garden.

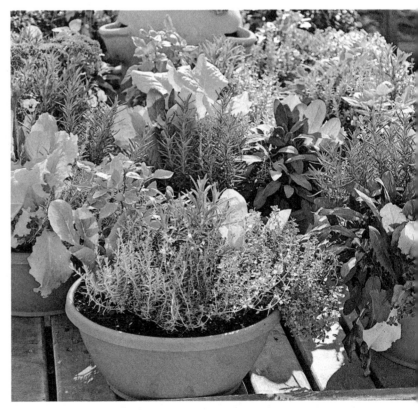

SEED SOURCING

One of the thrills of winter is getting the spring seed catalogs. Truly, as the polar vortex rages outside, I always seem to be tucked into the couch, cozy under a heavy blanket, reading about the hundreds of medicinal plant options that could be making their way into my summer rotation.

Although they help to make subzero temps more tolerable, these catalogs are also hugely helpful for general growing knowledge as well, because beyond the luscious descriptions, these catalogs—both in print and online—provide a wealth of information that can be used to plan a better garden strategy. When studying them, pay particular attention to these aspects:

- **Hardiness zone:** Shown in the accompanying chart (on pages 22 to 23), the United States is divided into plant hardiness zones that help growers and gardeners determine what's suitable for where they live, based on average annual minimum temperatures. Lower numbers mean the average annual temperatures are colder, and higher numbers mean the temperatures are more toasty. For example, Hawaii includes Zones 9 to 13, while Alaska includes Zones 1 to 4. Our farm is in Zone 4b. That means I choose herbs that grow with 4 as the minimum threshold—a plant catalog will specify "Zones 4 to 8" for instance—but I wouldn't pick an herb that thrives in a warmer zone, like those marked for "Zones 6 to 10." This all sounds like a middle school math problem, but the basic message is: know your zone (look on the map if you need to), and choose your seeds accordingly.
- **Light requirements:** Many medicinal plants prefer full sun, but some do better in partial shade. Knowing this information before ordering will help you plan your garden space more effectively.
- **Plant spacing:** This will help you determine whether you'll be putting in ten cilantro plants or just a few into a container by the walkway.
- **Days to maturity:** This is one of the most crucial pieces of info, because it can help you gauge when to expect harvest. Even with plants that regenerate, like many herbs do, I like to have a sense of the timeframe from seeding to harvest.
- **Soil and fertilization needs:** Many seed companies will provide acidity level information, so you'll know if you have to adjust pH levels.
- **Plant management:** Some seed companies do a fantastic job of providing tips on pests, diseases, harvesting, and even storage. Reading through these descriptions can feel like a college agriculture course sometimes, and I've walked away from a seed catalog reading session knowing about things like pirate bugs (not as adorable as they sound).
- **Container gardening suitable:** Because of the rising interest in indoor growing and container gardening outside, seed companies have started putting some great information on their websites. High Mowing Organic Seeds, for instance, has a nice online section about the topic, including suggested varieties, tips on growing, and a "seed collection" of ten packets that tend to do well in containers.
- **Pest issues:** Some seed companies are very helpful in describing pest problems that could strike your medicinal plants. Much like vegetable growing, each plant tends to have its own specific pest issue, which can be exacerbated by other challenges like drought. It's worth the time to do some research on pest problems and to investigate non-toxic solutions that can be implemented.

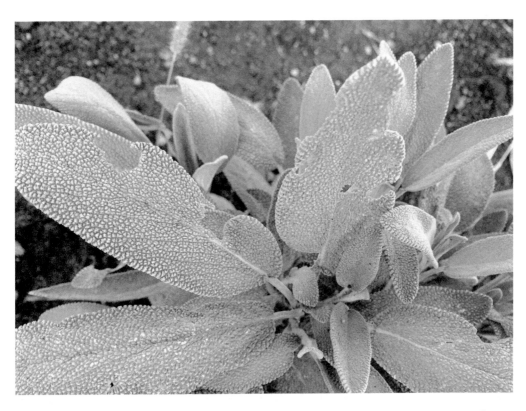

Sometimes, pest damage can be easy to spot, like these chewed-on leaves.

A quick note on organics here: because we own a farm that's been certified organic, we must buy organic seed, since that's part of the certification process. Beyond that, I'm a fan of organic growing, so even if we didn't have to use those types of seeds for Bossy Acres, I'd still buy them. I believe that organic practices lead to more sustainability, healthier soils, and a better agricultural system in general. Because of that, I think organic seeds are worth the extra cost that's usually involved in purchasing these seeds. You might opt for inexpensive, non-organic seeds instead, and that's fine, no judgment. But just know that all the cool kids these days are going organic.

Either way, make sure your seeds are coming from an established source, where you can get the type of growing information that you need. There have been many times that helpful family members have given me seeds from who-knows-where and they hand them over in little plastic bags. "This is celery," one of them will say. "Or it might be celeriac. I only marked it with 'cel' and it was a few years ago." That's the extent of the information I receive—they don't know the variety, growing timeframe, potential root depth, or anything else that help me make a decision in how I grow the plant. So, I usually just end up putting them in my backyard's raised beds, in a grab-bag experimental area that doesn't get much devotion or tending. Sometimes it works out, most times it doesn't.

No matter where you obtain your seeds, be sure to store them properly, in a plastic bin with a secure top. This will prevent numerous pest issues, and help to prolong the life of your seeds. For best results, use the seeds within a year or so, and sooner if possible. The older that seeds get, the less likely they are to germinate.

USDA PLANT HARDINESS ZONES

Average Annual Extreme
Minimum Temperature

1976-2005

Temp (F)	Zone	Temp (C)
-60 to -55	1a	-51.1 to -48.3
-55 to -50	1b	-48.3 to -45.6
-50 to -45	2a	-45.6 to -42.8
-45 to -40	2b	-42.8 to -40
-40 to -35	3a	-40 to -37.2
-35 to -30	3b	-37.2 to -34.4
-30 to -25	4a	-34.4 to -31.7
-25 to -20	4b	-31.7 to -28.9
-20 to -15	5a	-28.9 to -26.1
-15 to -10	5b	-26.1 to -23.3
-10 to -5	6a	-23.3 to -20.6
-5 to 0	6b	-20.6 to -17.8
0 to 5	7a	-17.8 to -15
5 to 10	7b	-15 to -12.2
10 to 15	8a	-12.2 to -9.4
15 to 20	8b	-9.4 to -6.7
20 to 25	9a	-6.7 to -3.9
25 to 30	9b	-3.9 to -1.1
30 to 35	10a	-1.1 to 1.7
35 to 40	10b	1.7 to 4.4
40 to 45	11a	4.4 to 7.2
45 to 50	11b	7.2 to 10
50 to 55	12a	10 to 12.8
55 to 60	12b	12.8 to 15.6
60 to 65	13a	15.6 to 18.3
65 to 70	13b	18.3 to 21.1

Alaska

Hawaii

USDA Plant Hardiness Zone Map,
2012. Agricultural Research Service,
U.S. Department of Agriculture. Access
from http://planthardiness.ars.usda.gov.

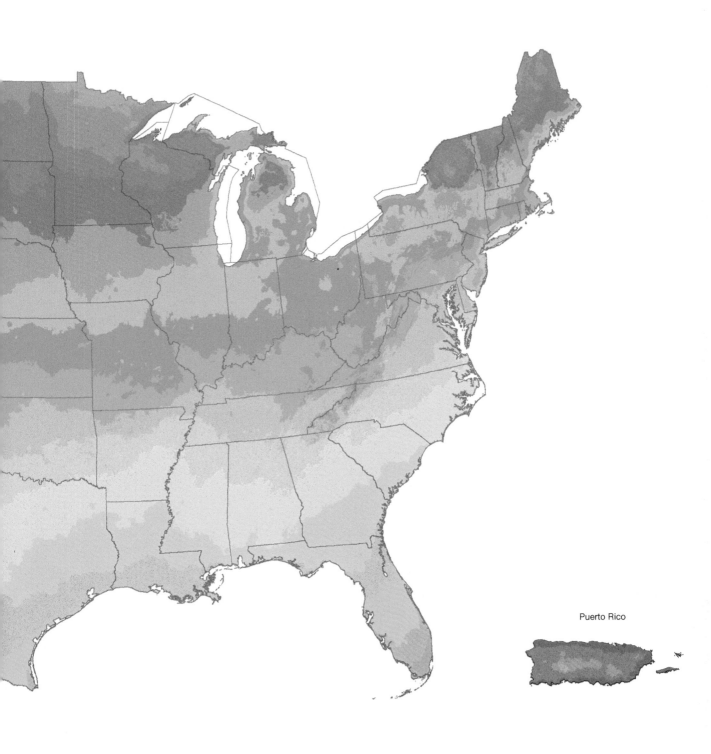

Puerto Rico

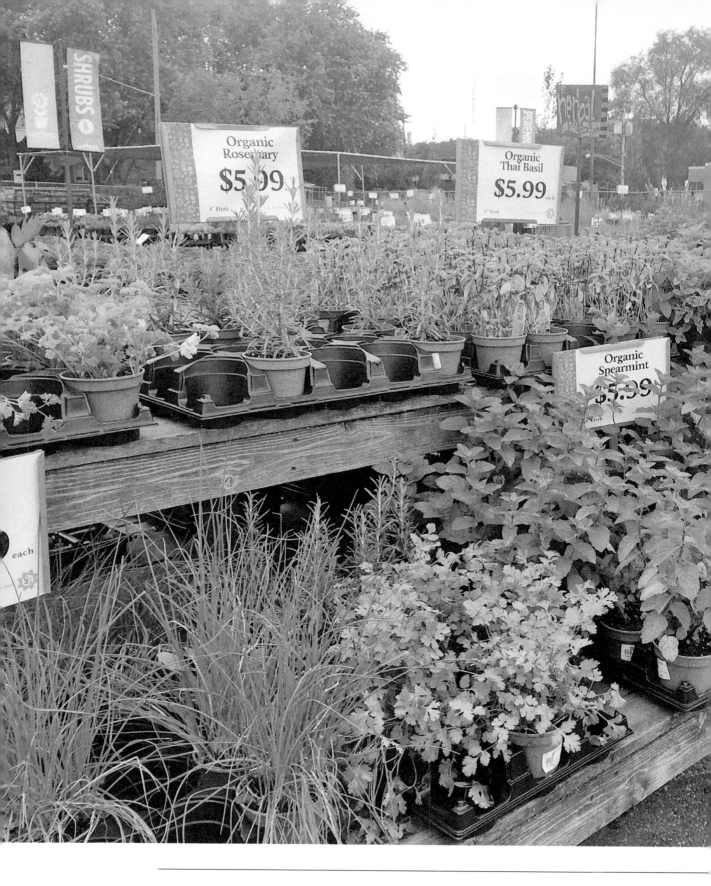

Organic
Rosemary
$5.99
4" Herb

Organic
Thai Basil
$5.99
4" Herb

Organic
Spearmint
$5.99
4" Herb

SHRUBS

herbal

each

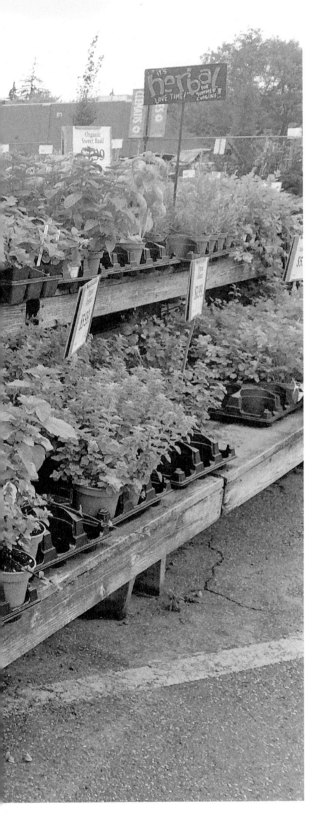

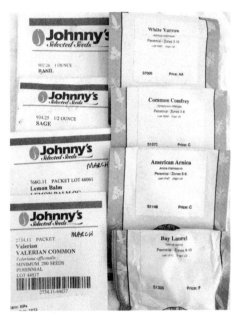

Opposite: Greenhouses and nurseries can be great places to find healthy plant starts, and many have organic options.

Seed packets usually have a nice amount of space on them for jotting down short notes.

Another handy tip: jot down notes right on the seed packet, including when the seeds were purchased. I use the packets for observations as well, noting what might be fast growing or whether a variety proved to be particularly good for tea, a decoction, a poultice, or other uses. It's very easy for me to lose track of notebooks, even when I try to store them with my growing supplies. But because I keep my empty seed packets in the same bin as my other seeds, I know where they are, and that one small packet will be rife with information, from both the seed company and my own experience.

TRANSPLANTS

Although there's a certain thrill with growing from seed, transplants might be more useful if you've had difficulty starting from seed before, or you just want to jumpstart your growing plan. If you're buying from a reliable source, transplants are a nice way to build your garden quickly.

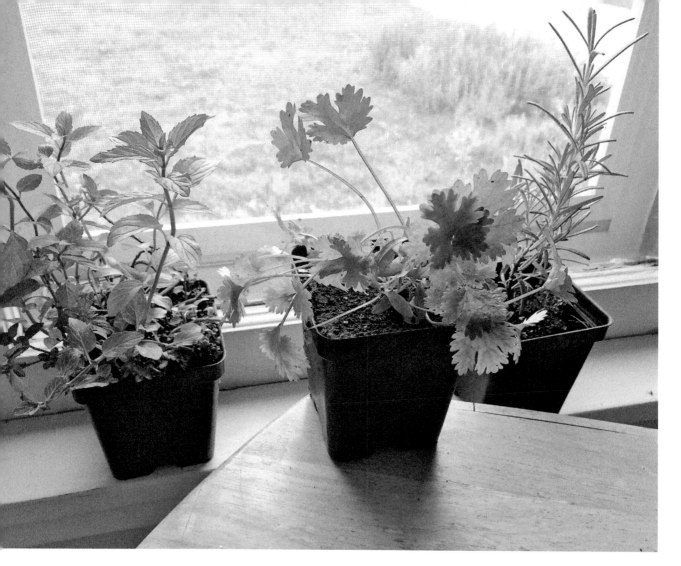

Even small windowsills can be handy for indoor growing options.

When buying transplants, be sure to inspect the plant thoroughly for any signs of pests or disease. A few dried leaves on the bottom usually aren't a problem, but if you see spotting, yellowing, or dryness on leaf edges, *choose another plant*. Also keep in mind that bigger isn't necessarily better. Many people opt for the largest transplants they can find, thinking that they're leapfrogging a month in the growing season—and sometimes it does work out that way. But in general, larger plants run the risk of transplant shock because they're more established and mature. Skip the behemoths and go for healthy, young transplants instead, which will be much easier to establish in a garden space.

INDOOR GROWING

Not to shill too heavily for my other book (*hey*, I have another book you can get!), but if you want to fill every available surface with green-and-leafy options, check out *Indoor Kitchen Gardening*. That covers all the picky little nuances of growing indoors, such as airflow, lighting, and container choices.

In general, though, many herbs are well suited for indoor growing, and several of the gardeners I know re-pot their outdoor garden herbs as the weather here gets crisp, so that they can extend the growing season indoors.

Some herbs, such as rosemary, oregano, thyme, and sage, propagate well if you take a cutting from an existing outdoor or indoor plant and prepare it for growth inside. If that's your strategy, simply cut a 4-inch section (measured from the tip of the stem/leaf toward the soil) and strip off about an inch or so of the lower leaves. Put the stem into a potting mix, such as vermiculite, and keep the mix somewhat moist as the plant establishes.

These plants like humidity, so cover with clear plastic or glass—letting light in, but trapping moisture—but don't let them get too hot from direct sunlight. Also, remove their covers occasionally or put them on a porch or "transitional" space to give them some air.

If you're bringing an entire plant inside, one that's already in a container, then be sure to make it a gradual process. For example, you might put the herb pot in a garage or porch for a week or two before placing it inside the house.

If using transplants from a garden store or farmers' market, then it's fine to bring them directly inside. The plants have already had a chance to be in an environment that's cozier than outside in the ground, and they're prepared for indoor growing.

Other medicinals, such as chamomile or berry plants, aren't exactly well-suited for indoor growing, and definitely any of the options from the Wild Yard Friends chapter are happier outside.

MAINTAINING GROWTH

Some medicinal plants, like calendula or elderberry, do well with regular watering but can withstand some dry days. Herbs, though, can be susceptible to overwatering, which can cause their roots to eventually rot. Even if you can avoid that fate, too much water may weaken the plant's immune system, causing disease or pests to take over. Each plant has different watering requirements, but in general, it's best to water when the soil *feels dry*, rather than keeping the herbs on a regular schedule in which you water automatically.

Another maintenance task is regular harvesting. This won't be too difficult, since you'll likely be using the plants often, but for those that you don't need immediately, it's a good idea to trim them back anyway and dry the harvested parts for later use. Not only does trimming help to keep a plant full and robust, but also the practice prevents bolting, which is the process by which a plant decides it's done for the season and "goes to seed" to prepare for the next. Bolting is often signaled by the growth of flowers, so if you're seeing those pop up, pinch the flowers off so you can extend the growing season.

In terms of fertilizer throughout the growing process, go easy. Many herbs, especially, like to be grown "lean," which means not too much food or water (although obviously that doesn't mean starve them of either). Too much fertilizer during the season tends to affect flavor, and can even reduce potency, since the herbs could have reduced essential oil as a result of the over-fertilization. That's good news for gardeners like me, who tend to like a little benign neglect in their growing practices.

In general, some medicinal plants can be very picky to grow, but for this book, I'm focusing on those that have thrived under my occasionally lazy care. Like any plant, medicinals will have to be tended, nurtured, and harvested, but the ones in this collection are all manageable for those who don't happen to be full-time gardeners. Let the fairy gardens begin.

STARTING SEEDS INDOORS

1. You can buy seed-starting tray kits at garden centers or home improvement stores. Usually you have to buy special seed-starting mix separately. This is a lightweight soilless mix made especially for starting seeds. Never use regular garden soil, as this soil can have fungi in it that kills emerging seedlings. Use a pencil to poke holes for the seeds in each section of the tray in which you'll plant the seeds.

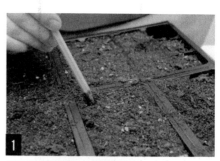

2. Plant one or two seeds per section of the seed-starting tray. Then water the soil until it is as moist as a wrung-out sponge. Depending upon the size of the sections in the seed-starting tray, you might or might not have to transplant plants into larger containers to grow before planting outside.

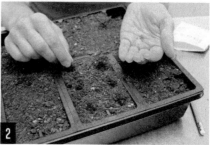

3. Cover the seed-starting tray with the plastic lid or with clear plastic cling wrap. This will keep the seeds moist. The top of the lid may become moist with condensation as the seeds begin to sprout. The condensation is a good thing, because it means you'll have to water the seeds less.

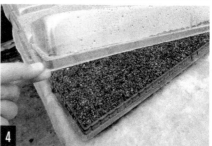

4. Check on the seeds as they're sprouting. If the top of the soil is dry, mist them with a spray bottle or very lightly water them. (Misting is better than watering because it is less likely to wash the delicate seedlings out of their spots in the trays.) Don't ever let seeds dry out while they're sprouting, or they'll die.

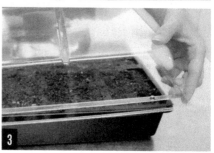

5. When seeds have two or more sets of "true leaves," you can transplant them into larger containers. Moving them up to 4-inch pots gives them room to grow and get larger and stronger before planting outside.

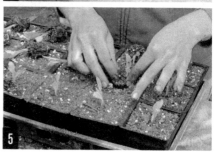

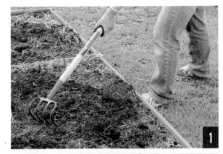

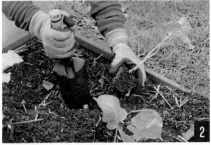

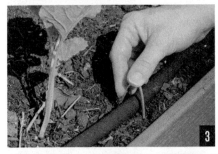

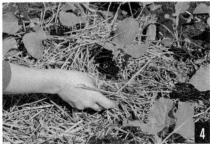

PLANTING TRANSPLANTS OUTDOORS

1. Before planting anything in the garden, get some worm castings (worm poop), mushroom compost, or composted cow manure to rake into the soil. Spread a 1-inch layer on top of the soil and use a four-tine claw to work it in.

2. Once the soil is prepared, set out the plants according to spacing instructions on the plant tag. Broccoli, cabbage, and kale plants need 12 to 18 inches of space between them. Lettuce only needs 8 inches of space between plants.

3. After you've planted everything, water each plant by placing the water breaker on the hose at the base of each plant and counting to ten. To make quick work of watering, put a soaker hose around your plants to water them. You can snake the hose in and out of rows and use wire pins called sod staples to hold down the hose. If the hose is in the middle of two rows, the water from it will reach plants on each side of the hose.

4. Spread mulch around the vegetable transplants. If you live in a warmer area, this will help keep water in the soil during those hot, Indian summer fall days. In cooler areas, the mulch acts to insulate the vegetables, helping them stay warmer longer into the fall. Straw is good for vegetable gardens because it is lightweight. Most garden centers and home improvement stores sell bales of wheat straw. Just ask for it if you don't see it.

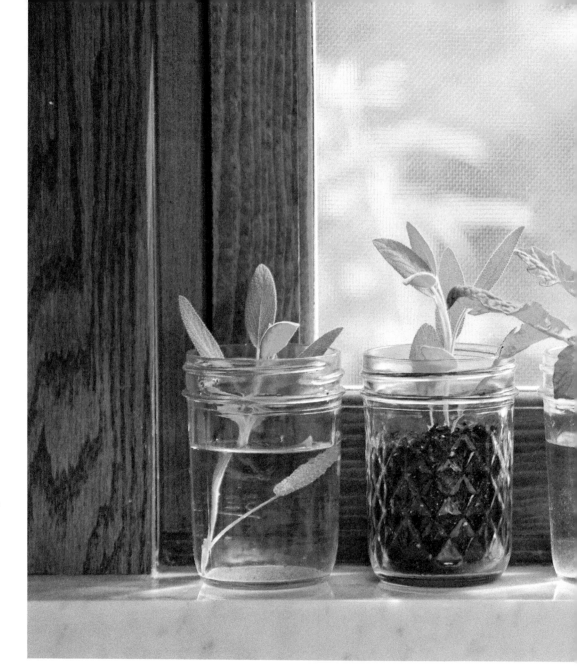

You can't do better than natural sunshine when it comes to providing a light source for starting and growing your edible indoor garden plants. But do be aware that too much sunlight will damage some of the more delicate plants.

ROOM TO GROW

Here's some bad news: you can't grow twenty different kinds of herbs on a 3-foot space in a kitchen. Believe me, I wish someone had told me that a few years ago.

Like plants out in a field or in an outdoor raised bed, indoor plants need space apart from each other to stretch out. With the exception of microgreens and shoots, which are harvested during the first stage of growth and don't need ample room to expand, most indoor plants benefit from at least some breathing room. Herbs and many types of vegetables can be cozy, but they shouldn't be crowded.

When picking your growing spot and making a plan, create a rough sketch of where each pot or container will go, to give yourself a visual representation of your indoor garden. When it begins to

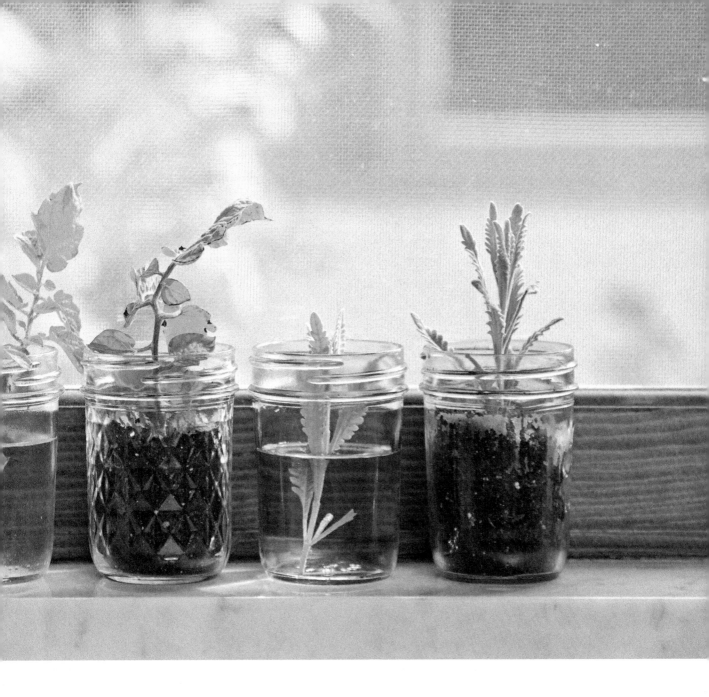

feel like a game of Tetris, consider scaling back on the number of plants in favor of giving the top contenders a better shot at growth.

If you plant your in-home garden near a water source, such as the kitchen sink, you'll have the option of bringing the plants to water. The main reason this is preferable is that it eliminates the risk of spilling water all around the plants set up throughout the home.

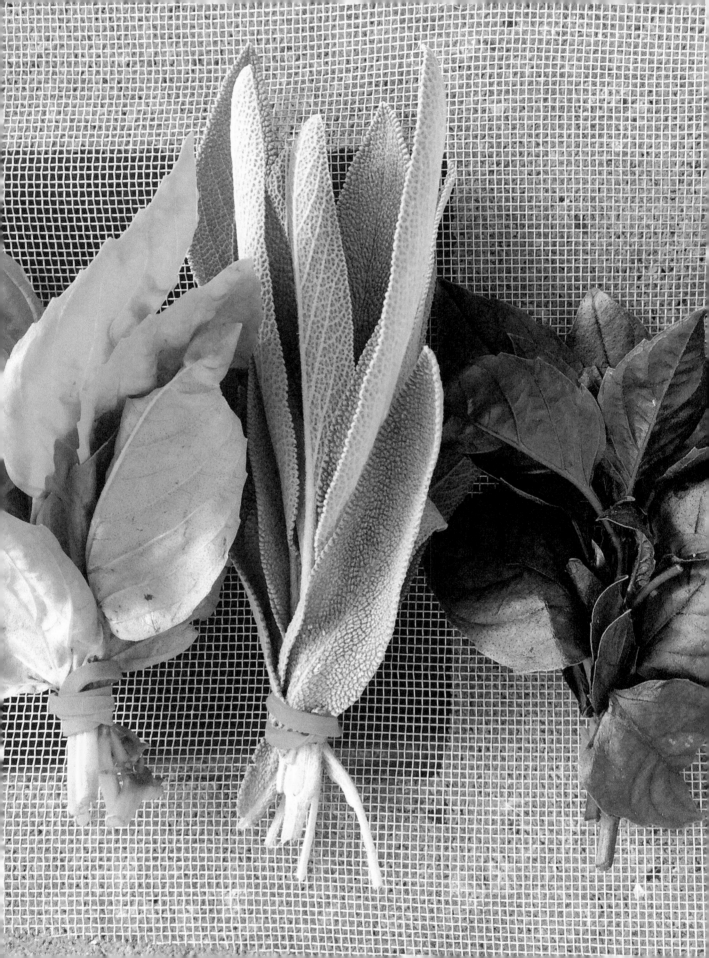

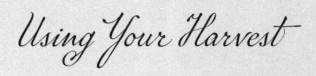

TWO

Using Your Harvest

Growing medicinal plants can be deeply satisfying, but when you're able to utilize those herbs in meaningful ways, then they truly become therapeutic marvels.

Fortunately, most preparations aren't complex, and can be done with what you already have on hand. In other cases, a few modest purchases (such as a spice grinder and dark-colored jars) will greatly expand your homegrown medicine cabinet. Putting equipment like a mortar and pestle on the kitchen counter can be a nice reminder to make the most of a harvest.

Often, I find that preparing remedies has a therapeutic effect in itself, since many of those moments involve slowing down, collecting ingredients like honey or olive oil, and laying out plant components in front of me. Dried leaves, bits of root or bark, or a smattering of flower petals are spread out in front of me, and no matter how frantic my day has been, creating a tea or infusion is an instant downshift.

I've also been gratified to see how well these remedies work. Even simple ones, like sipping on a "happy tummy" tea or making a warm poultice, seem to speed healing faster than anticipated.

Much like creating a growing space, planning for remedies is the key for success. Clear off part of a counter, make room on a bookshelf, or set aside a cool dry part of a cupboard and designate that as your new medicine space.

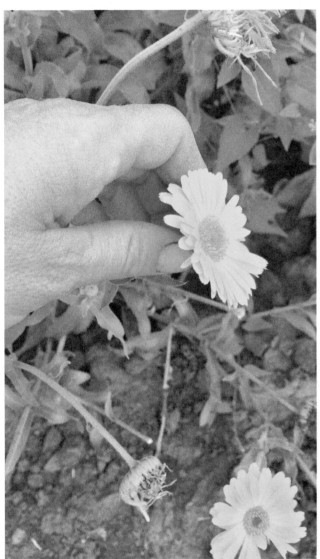
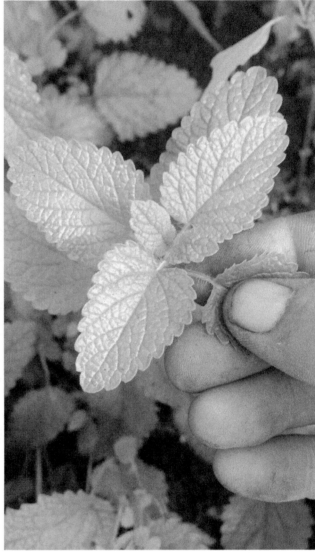

HARVESTING BASICS

Harvesting flowers is usually very simple, you just pluck the blooms at the top of the stem.

When plucking leaves, make sure to choose leaves that have good color and are free of white or brown spots.

Flowers and leaves: Most of the time, harvesting is as simple as plucking a flower or leaf from the plant. When making those selections, be sure to first examine what you're about to harvest, to doublecheck that there are no plant issues, such as white or brown spots on the leaves, whitish coating under a leaf, or a sickly looking bloom with pale coloring. Herbal remedies are at their most efficacious when a healthy plant is used, and trying to create a tea or decoction from an unhealthy plant can result in sour or bitter taste or a less-effective treatment.

Bark: There are some plants that hold medicinal properties in the bark—well-known examples include willow bark, slippery elm, and cramp bark, but there are many others. To harvest from

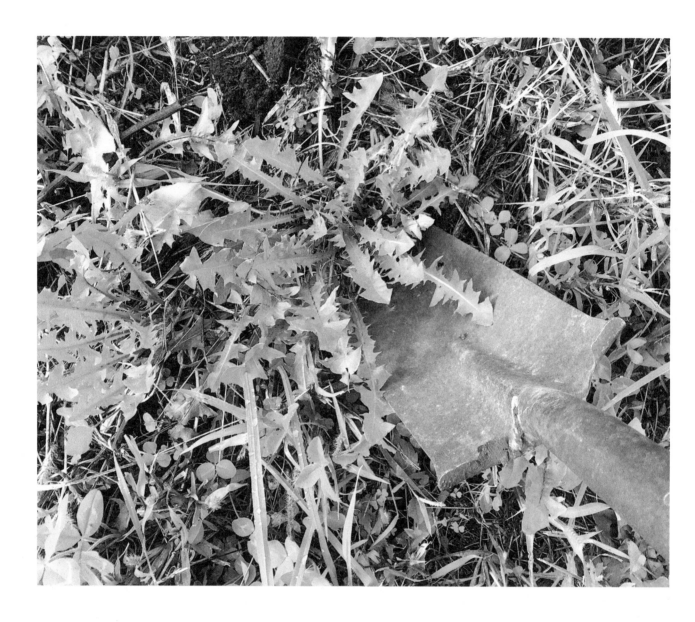

younger trees and plants, strip the bark off young branches in the spring, when they haven't yet gotten tough from a long growing season. For older plants, chose a part that's away from the central trunk or main section, since you don't want to negatively affect the plant's growth. Some bark can be used immediately, but in general, you'll want to dry it so it can store for longer.

Roots: When an herbal remedy involves using a plant's roots, it's usually best to harvest in the fall, particularly October or November, after the ground plants have either faded or died back completely with a few frosts. This is when plants bring their energy away from the leaves, blooms, and fruit and focus instead on winter storage, which means that the roots will have more potency. There are some

When harvesting roots, use a small shovel so you don't have to displace much soil.

Small herb bundles for drying can be used for decorative effect as well as utility.

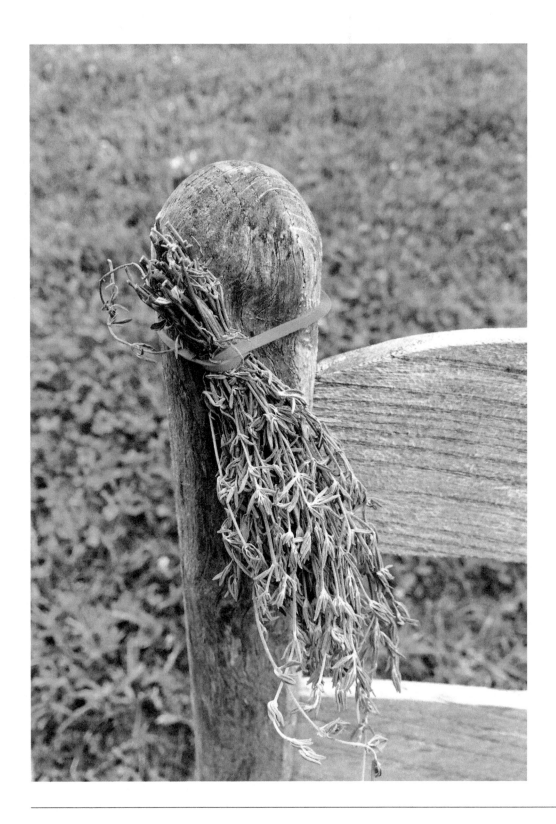

exceptions, such as dandelion, but in general, aim to harvest roots in the autumn and store them, dried, over the winter months. When harvesting, take only what you plan to use, leaving the majority of the roots in the ground so the plant can continue with its winter hibernation. Be sure to cover the area where you dug, otherwise the other roots may be exposed to cold, affecting a plant's health.

PREPARING REMEDIES

Once you have your leaves, flowers, bark, or roots, there are just a couple ways you can prepare them. First, simply plan to use them fresh, and make sure to create whatever topical or internal remedy you prefer as soon as possible after harvesting, to increase potency.

For other remedies or long-term storage, though, you'll want to dry the plant sections. This

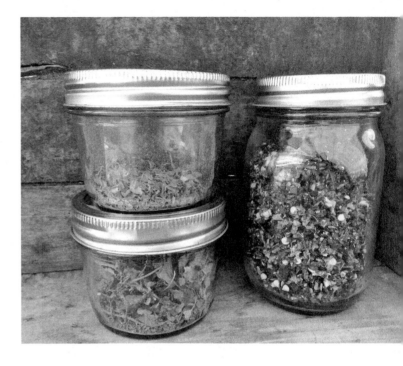

Canning jars are ideal for storing your preparations.

ensures that mold doesn't become a factor, which would thwart all your good intentions. I usually dry leaves and flowers on a clean mesh screen—plastic, coated metal, or sometimes cheesecloth stretched tight—and leave them in a dry and well-ventilated area. A garage with an open door works well, as long as it's not dusty, or if you have a breezy attic space (particularly with rafters), that tends to be ideal as well.

Create bundles of herbs by tying the stems and hanging so the stem side is up; this concentrates the active properties downward, into the blooms and leaves. For roots and bark, leave on the mesh surface for an extended time, up to a few years for particularly slow-drying herbs, and test for "doneness" by breaking a section off. It should snap easily, like a dried twig for kindling. If it bends instead, extend the drying process.

When the components are dry, store them in airtight jars, and ideally in colored jars. You can often find dark brown or blue jars, and these are best since they prevent any light from affecting the herbs inside. Put the jars inside a cupboard or closet where they won't be too humid; usually a basement space works well.

CULINARY AND INTERNAL USES

When using medicinal plants for maladies like gastrointestinal distress, insomnia, menstrual issues, or colds, you have the option of using fresh leaves and flowers, or utilizing the dried components you've been storing. With culinary preparations, I usually prefer fresh plants if they're available, since I love the pop of flavor that comes with throwing some just-harvested basil or lemon balm on a dish, but that technique doesn't work well in a Minnesota winter. Instead, I employ these strategies:

Keeping some supplies on hand—like a spice grinder, mortar and pestle, and cheesecloth—can be very useful.

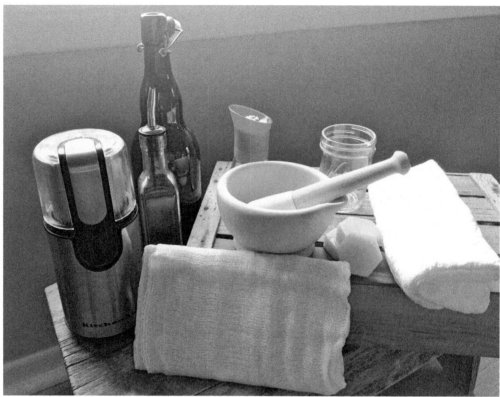

Left: Tea bags can be found in several sizes and are easy to reuse.

Right: Pouring alcohol into your herbs or dried plant parts can keep them potent for years.

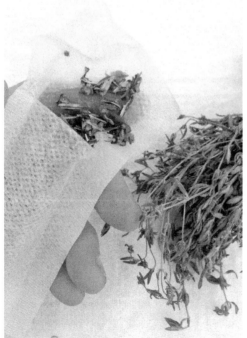

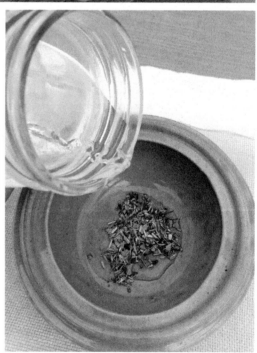

Tea or infusion: This tends to be the go-to method, because it's easy and quick. Simply take dried or fresh leaves and flowers, put in a cup or bowl, and pour just-boiled water over the plant parts.

Steeping (which means letting the plant components sit in the water) time depends on the herbal preparation. For example, I've found that mint gets bitter if steeped for too long, but chamomile can withstand a longer steep time of up to 10 minutes. To use, just strain the liquid and drink.

Decoction: For tougher plant parts, such as roots and bark, you'll need a more intense method of extracting the vital components, and a decoction works well for that. Put plant parts in a pot (ideally enamel, since metal can make herbs go wonky), bring to a boil, and then reduce to a simmer.

Cook for an hour so the liquid reduces. Then strain it through cheesecloth or a fine-meshed sieve into a heatproof jar or bowl, like a Mason jar or Pyrex container, and allow it to cool before using.

Tincture: A stellar preparation method, tinctures involve steeping a plant part in alcohol, usually vodka since it contains the least impurities. You place fresh or dried leaves, flowers, or roots into a clean jar and add a mix of two-thirds vodka to one-third water. In terms of quantity, you want the parts to be able to move freely when shaking the jar, but you can still put in a significant amount.

For two weeks of a tincture, shake the jar gently every day, and store in a cool, dark place. After a couple weeks, strain the liquid through cheesecloth or muslin into a new, clean bottle, preferably one that's brown or blue colored, so the properties aren't affected by light. You can store the resulting liquid for a few years.

In some cases, you can simply leave the plant parts in the vodka indefinitely. I have a jar of Solomon's seal roots that has served me well through several farm seasons, since I use only a few drops on sore muscles.

Essential oil creation: Concentrating the medicinal properties of a plant, essential oils are what you usually find in any co-op or natural foods store. In their little brown bottles, complete with droppers that allow for precise dosages, the oils are highly useful, but not very easy to make at home unless you build or buy a still. If you're up for the project—which tends to feel like making moonshine—then embark on that journey, but I much prefer simple strategies that don't require a few hundred dollars in upfront costs.

You can also use a solvent, such as hexane, to extract the oil and employ another solvent, usually ethyl alcohol, to create the oil, but distillation is still involved. In this book, we focus on modest-scale medicinal plant growing, so we'll be skipping homegrown distillation in favor of simple remedy creation. But hey, if you're already making moonshine, then visit www.essential-oil-mama.com and follow her helpful advice for essential oil creation. However, even she admits that distillation is an art, and homemade essential oils tend to be less useful than professionally produced, therapeutic-grade essential oils.

TOPICAL PREPARATIONS

Over the past few years, I've come to rely on herbs almost exclusively for any kind of external issue—dry skin, chapped lips, bruises, minor scrapes, splinters, insect bites, bee stings, rashes, and other irritations. Preparations for these don't take long, and they often produce immediate relief. Also, utilizing a tactic like a poultice or a compress is relaxing, because who doesn't like a touch of spa-level treatment? Try these:

Poultice: Blend fresh or dried leaves or flowers with a small amount of just-boiled water, only enough to dampen the plant components. This should create a thick paste that can be spread directly on the skin while it's still warm. Wrap clean gauze over the paste and leave for a few hours, then repeat if necessary.

Compress: Often considered less messy than a poultice, a compress still has the same general idea of putting herbs on the skin and using heat to release their properties. For a compress, first make an infusion or decoction of a the plant parts, then soak a piece of clean gauze or cloth in the liquid. Squeeze out any excess liquid, and then place the compress against the skin. Usually, I place a warm towel over the compress to make the treatment more soothing, but it's not mandatory for deriving benefits from the plants.

A mortar and pestle can be handy for grinding dried herbs quickly.

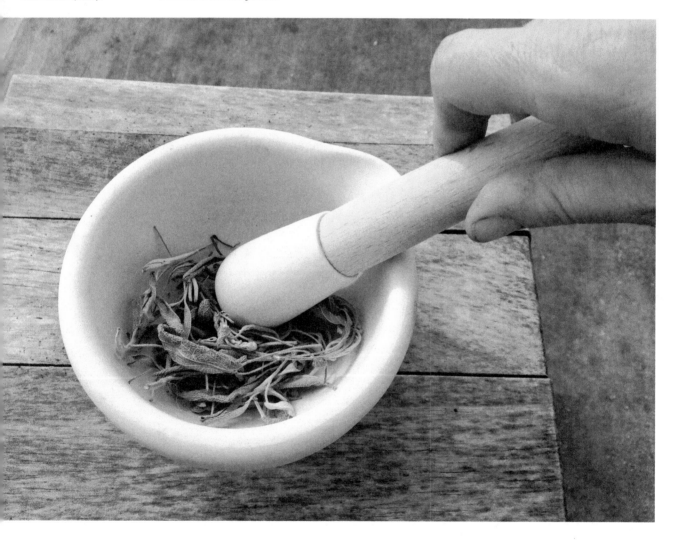

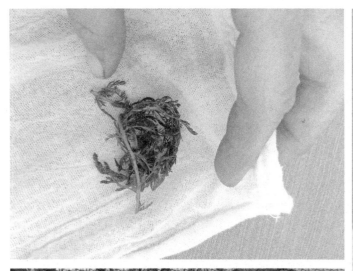

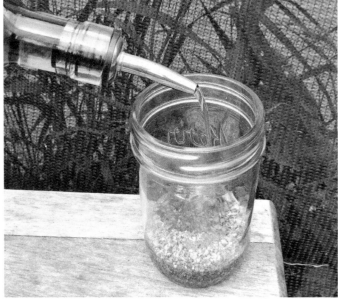

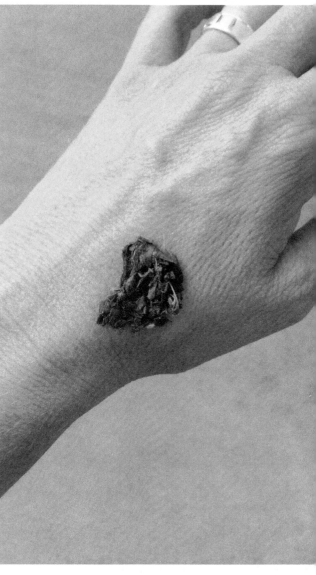

Infused oil: There are a couple methods for making infused oil, but the easiest is to place dried or fresh plant parts (usually leaves or flowers) into a jar and fill with olive oil to about 1 inch from the top of whatever jar or bottle you're using. Seal the container and place in a sunny, warm window so the sunlight can work some magic to break down the plant parts.

Shake the jar at least once per day to keep all the components from settling on the bottom, and after a few weeks, strain the mixture and bottle into a new container. Infused oil can also be used for cooking, and imparts quite a bit of flavor to dishes with just a light drizzle.

Salve: The least messy of all, a salve can be very helpful for using medicinal treatments while moisturizing and nourishing the skin. Just take your infused oil and choose a base for the salve—

Top left: Steeped herbs being placed in a clean piece of cheesecloth to use as a poultice.

Bottom left: Putting dried plant parts together with olive oil, for cooking or medicinal preparations.

Above: Chewed plantain leaves placed directly on an insect bite reduces itching and swelling.

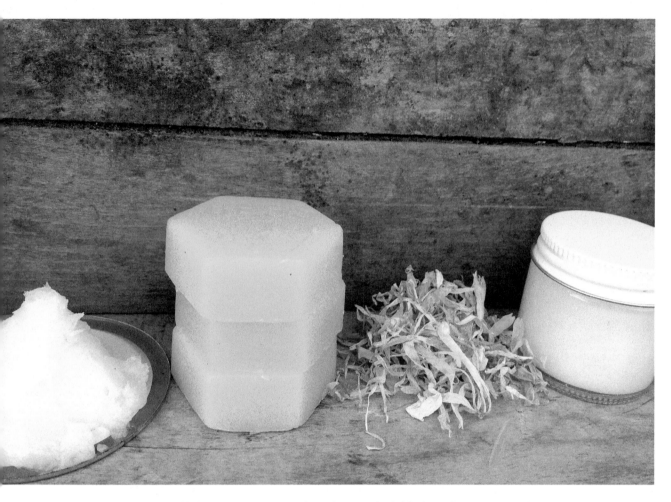

Ingredients for a balm might include coconut oil, beeswax, dried petals, and lotion.

usually beeswax or coconut oil—and essential oils like lavender if you want the mix to have a pleasant fragrance. Put about 1 ounce of your base and 8 ounces of infused oil into a double boiler to prevent scorching and gently warm over low heat until they all fuse together. Be sure to keep the heat very low and definitely *don't* boil, which can cause the olive oil to oxidize.

When it's still warm, pour into small tins or glass jars, and let cool completely before storing in a cool place. Although the salves will be in a solid state, they melt easily with body heat. Medicinals that work particularly well for salves include calendula, arnica, burdock root, and comfrey. If you're dealing with sore muscles, a cayenne pepper salve can be a nice choice, similar to over-the-counter treatments that warm the skin on contact.

RESEARCH, RESEARCH, RESEARCH

Finally, a note about awareness: although medicinal plants have been used successfully for thousands of years, helping millions of people, that certainly doesn't mean every plant is safe for any condition. Some medicinals conflict in significant ways with prescription medicine, and even with one another.

For instance, the interactions with medications and St. John's wort have been so profound that France has banned all use of products containing the herb. Damiana, used to treat depression, sexual problems, and low energy, has been shown to decrease blood sugar, which is usually a great thing, unless you're taking diabetes medicine that also lowers blood sugar levels. There are numerous other examples of interactions that could put people at risk, including use of yarrow (see "Harvest & Store" section of the yarrow profile), wormwood, ginko, and black cohosh.

In addition to interactions, some herbs have simply been proven to have negative effects after several studies were undertaken. Most notably, comfrey used to be recommended as a tea—I own one herbal guide from 1983 that recommends drinking three cups of it per day—but research has shown such a high level of toxicity to the liver that herbalists now warn that you shouldn't even use it on scrapes because it can get into your system that way.

So, even with history and ancient healing as our guide, I believe that scientific research certainly has a place in contemporary herbal medicine. That's why I've included research study citations in each chapter, to indicate a plant's efficacy, and to encourage you to do your own research when it comes to preparations. If you're taking prescriptions or regularly use over-the-counter medication, investigate whether there have been any warnings in terms of interactions with specific plants that you're interested in trying.

If your medical doctor is open to talking to about herbal complements to any maladies, have a discussion about potential effects, and consult with your holistic physician about interactions with vitamins and supplements. Most of all, listen to your gut (sometimes literally). If a medicinal isn't working for you, or makes you feel off in any way, discontinue use immediately. As much as we all love optimism and good intentions, they shouldn't override someone's instincts about what feels healthy and what doesn't.

ENJOY THE ADVENTURE

With all of the caveats about drug-and-herb interactions aside, the fact is that medicinal plants can be a stellar addition to your health and wellness plan. They're incredibly fun to grow, and when your hands smell like cilantro and calendula after a day of harvesting, the stress tends to melt away on its own.

So, make your growing and preparation into an adventure instead of into more to-do list items that seem to expand like weeds. With very simple, one-ingredient remedies, it's easy to get started with using a few plants at a time, and thanks to tasty favorites like basil and mint, you can find yourself mixing up your own spice blends like a culinary school valedictorian. Plus, you'll have a cabinet full of medicinal options when it comes to common maladies, thanks to your genius with salves, decoctions, tinctures, and teas.

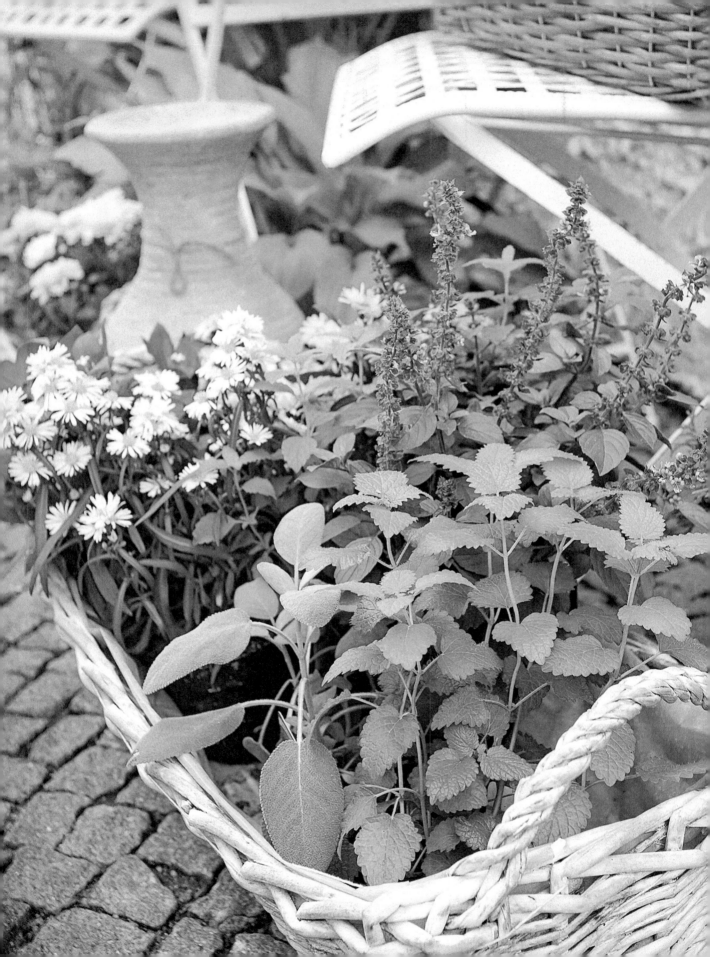

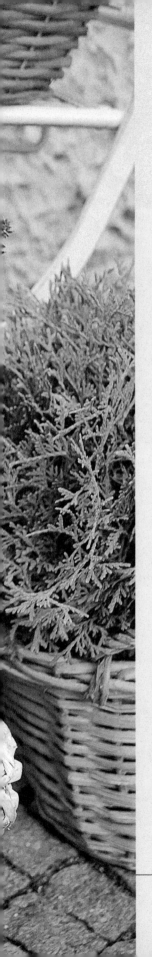

THREE

Kitchen Garden Herbs

When many people think about medicinal herbs, they tend to envision varieties that sound like they might pop up in a Victorian novel: blackwort, centaury, damiana, feverfew, juniperus, and perhaps the best named of all, false unicorn.

While there are plenty of those types of herbs in use, and we'll cover some charmingly named ones in the next section, there's also a wealth of medicinal options that come from a kitchen garden and wouldn't be out of place on a spice rack.

Herbs like sage, peppermint, oregano, and other culinary options give zip and flavor to meals, but they also have health benefits. Integrating these into your medicinal mix is easy, especially since they're so tasty. Plus, finding medicinal uses helps to conquer the "too many herbs" issue when a whole garden is ready for harvest.

On our farm, I often sample these herbs throughout the day for a quick pick-me-up in the middle of harvesting or planting. My pockets always seem to have a few leaves of Thai basil or spearmint, so I can pop them into my mouth the same way other people might reach for gum.

Best of all, growing culinary herbs is generally simple, depending on plant hardiness zone (see the book's introduction for a chart of zones). You can have a small windowbox of favorite herbs, or an expansive backyard garden that would make any chef pale with envy. So, let's get growing.

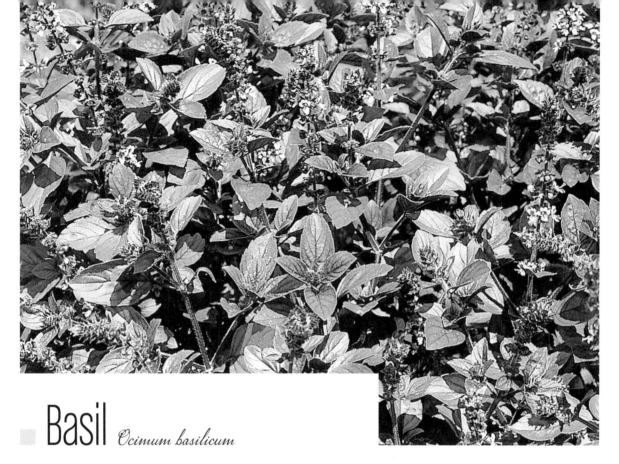

Basil *Ocimum basilicum*

Basil boasts a rich history of medicinal as well as culinary uses. In addition to being utilized worldwide for flavoring sauces, soups, and killer pesto, basil has been used for Ayurvedic medicine, liqueurs, and traditional Chinese medicine. Most often, it's used for treating the digestive system, although in some parts of the world, like Africa, basil also lends itself to kidney treatments and fever reduction. It's been said to boost libido, clear the head during a cold, and improve concentration. Theories abound as to basil's origins, and some sources place its birthplace as Southeast Asia while others believe it's Africa. Either way, it arrived in Europe through the Middle East and landed first in Italy. From there, basil spread across the planet, although the United States has become one of the largest producers.

Basil leaf can impart sedative, diuretic, and antiseptic properties. The herb is safe for children, and can even hurry chicken pox through the body.

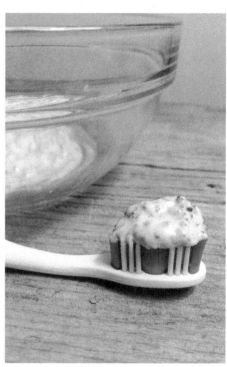

Just a small amount of basil can have big benefits.

Here are a few ideas for your Rx/medicinal preparations:

- Chew on fresh leaves to reduce the impact of infections in the mouth, alleviate cold symptoms, or loosen mucus in the respiratory system.
- Grind up dried leaves into a powder and add to toothpaste to freshen breath and reduce bacteria.
- Use dried leaves in a tea to alleviate headaches, act as a calmative for insomnia, or lessen menstruation pain.
- Put chewed-up leaves on insect stings to reduce itching, pain, and inflammation.
- Boil fresh leaves and strain, then drink to lower fevers; this method is especially useful if you mix in cardamom or feverfew.

PLANT·GROW·HARVEST·USE

Basil isn't particularly frost resistant, so it tends to be best in warmer climates, but can truly be grown almost anywhere. It does well with abundant sunshine, and in general, it's a good choice for any region because it can be brought inside if temps begin dropping in fall.

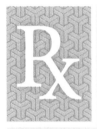

MEDICINE CABINET

Basil provides notable potential health benefits, particularly if used in essential oil form. In the academic journal *Food Chemistry*, researchers found high levels of antioxidants in basil oil, and some effectiveness as an antimicrobial and antibacterial remedy.

Reduce inflammation and swelling

A study presented at the Royal Pharmaceutical Society's annual event revealed that "extracts of *O. tenuiflorm* (Holy basil) were shown to reduce swelling by up to 73 percent 24 hours after treatment."[1]

Anti-aging properties

According to research, basil can help prevent the harmful effects of aging. Holy basil extract was effective at killing off harmful molecules and preventing damage caused by some free radicals in the liver, brain, and heart.[2]

Rich in antioxidants

Results of a study published in the *Journal of Advanced Pharmacy Education & Research* showed that ethanol extract *Ocimum basilicum* had more antioxidant activity than standard antioxidants.[3]

1 http://www.hort.purdue.edu/newcrop/ncnu02/v5-575.html

2 Prakash P, Gupta N. Therapeutic uses of Ocimum sanctum Linn (Tulsi) with a note on eugenol and its pharmacological actions: a short review. *Indian Journal Physiol*. Pharmacol 2005; 49: 125-131

3. http://www.japer.in/Issue/Issu%202%20august/18.pdf

Sun: Six to eight hours per day

Shade: Some shade tolerance, especially in hotter climates

Soil: Well-drained, loosened soil

Fertilizer: Apply some around base every few weeks, particularly if plants are struggling. Does well with compost, bloodmeal, or cottonseed meal

Pests: Aphids, slugs, or beetles, but these tend to be minimal

Water: Regularly, depending on soil dryness

Grow Indoors? Yes

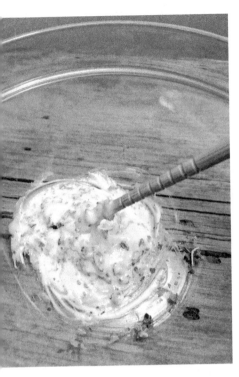

Basil can be ground up and mixed with toothpaste to freshen breath and reduce bacteria.

VARIETIES You're likely to think first of sweet basil (like Genovese or Italian), the variety that appears in grocery stores and pasta dishes, but there are numerous options, and each boasts distinctive characteristics in terms of flavor. Basic medicinal properties are fairly consistent across varieties (although Holy basil has the most history as a healing herb), so choose based on taste preferences.

- **Thai basil:** has such a strong anise flavor that it's sometimes called "licorice basil"
- **Holy basil:** also known as Tulsi; very popular in India and Thailand, where it's treasured for its medicinal properties; spicy taste and slightly fuzzy leaves; a blend of minty and basil flavors
- **Italian large leaf basil:** the classic sweet basil used most frequently in cooking; large green leaves; has a sweet taste that goes well with Italian dishes
- **Napoletano:** similar in flavor to the Italian variety, but with huge leaves that resemble lettuce; needs plenty of room for growth
- **Purple basil:** has several varieties like Purple Ruffles, Dark Opal, Red Rubin, and Amethyst; all have a luscious, deep purple color
- **Lemon basil:** petite but very flavorful; has a citrus undertone that makes it perfect for teas

PLANT Basil does well started indoors and then transplanted outside, so if you have a greenhouse space, that's ideal. However, even a kitchen windowsill will work. Place seeds in a tray or small individual pots, and water well. When starting seeds, depending on the warmth of the room, germination should take about five to ten days, but can be accelerated by using a germination mat— these are like plant heating pads that don't scorch the roots but keep the plant cozy as it establishes. Once basil is 3 to 5 inches tall, transplant outdoors or into a large container, if that's where you plan to grow it. Or, transplant into a bigger pot for indoor growing so the roots have more room to expand.

Many gardeners buy transplants rather than starting from seed, and this can be a stellar jumpstart, especially since basil is easily obtained from commercial growers. Look for hearty, well-established plants that have both established (mature) and new leaves. One advantage to buying transplants is that they've already been "hardened" (adapted) to outside temperatures, so they can be transplanted right away.

Aim for loose, well-drained soil in either outdoor or indoor plantings. If growing inside, make sure that the pot can drain properly—avoid letting the plant sit in water—so that the roots stay dry. If planting outside, be sure to loosen the soil around the transplant and avoid compaction when securing it in its new home.

Basil thrives most at around 80 degrees Fahrenheit, and needs around six to eight hours of sunshine per day; those living in hotter places should consider planting where there's some shade at least part of the day.

GROW Once basil plants are established and thriving, water the soil rather than the leaves, to prevent disease or mildew. You can fertilize every few weeks; basil does well with compost, bloodmeal, or cottonseed meal. If the plants seem hearty, though, you're fine skipping this step unless they seem to be struggling through slow growth or overly drooping leaves.

Aphids or beetles can sometimes be a problem, and you'll see either the insects themselves, or leaves that are bitten with little holes or chewed along the edges. If that's an issue, consider using a product like a fabric rowcover such as Reemay. This is a very lightweight fabric that lets sunshine and rain come through, but can keep pests out.

Depending on weather or indoor temperatures—hotter temps make basil grow faster—basil will begin flowering within a few weeks of maturity. Since this is a signal to the plant that its time is coming to an end, just snip off the flowers to prolong growth. Done often enough, this simple technique can extend your basil-growing season significantly.

Most varieties take about 60 to 75 days from planting to maturity, although you can harvest along the way if the plant is becoming well-established.

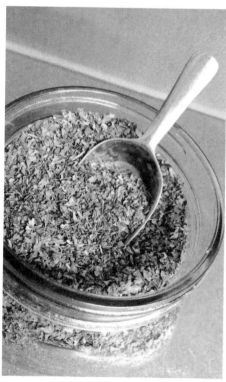

Store dried basil in tightly sealed canning jars.

HARVEST & STORE Basil does best with frequent harvesting. Leave the smallest top leaves alone and pluck off larger leaves to encourage growth and create a stronger, heartier plant. Often, I've stripped a plant down to almost nothing except a few leaves of new growth, to come back in a week or so to find it lush again. For best results, pluck off the leaves rather than cutting them. Store these ways:

Fresh: this is the best method for cooking and salads, since basil has such an intense, pleasant flavor. Just chop or tear the leaves.

Dry: you can use a food dehydrator, but I tend to get good results by simply placing the leaves on a mesh screen in a well-ventilated area like my porch. If you worry about pests or dust, lightly cover the leaves with Reemay or other lightweight fabric that allows for air circulation.

Concentrated: create an oil (see Using Your Harvest chapter, page 41 for info on infused oils) that can be used in a bath, daubed on insect bites, or even used in a salad dressing.

NUTRITIONAL VALUE OF BASIL

per 100 g (3.5 oz)

Basil is rich in vitamin A, vitamin K, vitamin C, magnesium, iron, potassium, and calcium.

Energy	94 kJ (22 kcal)
Carbohydrates	2.65 g
Dietary fiber	1.6 g
Fat	0.64 g
Protein	3.15 g
Water	92.06 g
Vitamin A	264 g
Thiamine	0.034 g
Riboflavin	0.076 g
Niacin	0.902 g
Vitamin B$_6$	0.155 g
Folate	68 g
Choline	11.4 mg
Vitamin C	18.0 mg
Vitamin E	0.80 mg
Vitamin K	414.8 g
Calcium	177 mg
Iron	3.17 mg
Magnesium	64 mg
Manganese	1.148 mg
Phosphorus	56 mg
Potassium	295 mg
Sodium	4 mg
Zinc	0.81 mg

Source: USDA Nutrient Database

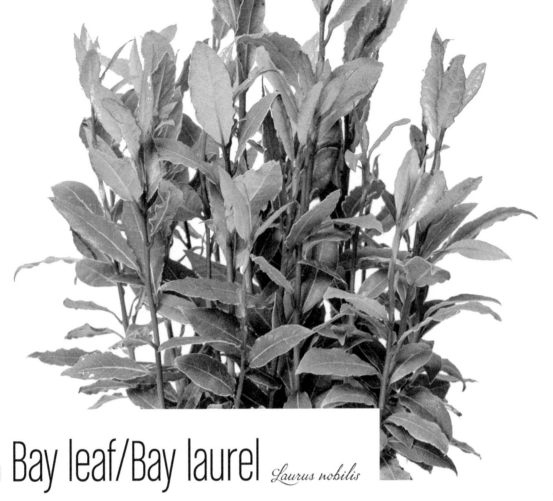

Bay leaf/Bay laurel *Laurus nobilis*

Even when I was brewing teas with wild-growing nettles and eating lamb's quarter salads (see the Wild Yard Friends chapter for info on both of these herbal standouts), I still didn't see bay leaf as anything more than the inedible seasoning addition that got thrown into soups and stews. Now I'm humbled by that dismissal. Bay leaf has a long and rich history, both for its health properties and its metaphorical power. The Greeks and Romans believed the herb symbolized peace, wisdom, and honor, and the leaves were woven into wreaths that crowned athletes and royalty. Originating in Asia Minor, the leaves are now one of the most widely used herbs throughout North America and Europe, thanks to their distinctive flavor, unique fragrance, and distinctive health properties.

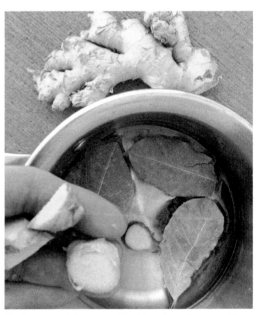

Bay leaves and ginger combined in a decoction can make a fragrant bath addition.

Legend notes that the Delphi princess in ancient Greece inhaled smoldering bay leaves in order to hear Apollo's prophecies, so it's only natural that bay is recommended for some less-than-medicinal purposes, like encouraging prophetic dreams (just tuck some under your pillow) or increasing psychic ability by inhaling smoke from a bay smudge. But the herb has wellness uses, especially for pain relief and digestion issues.

Here are a few ideas for your Rx/medicinal preparations:

- For a headache or migraine, lightly steam a few bay leaves—the steam setting of an iron works well—and then rest with the warm leaves on your forehead for at least half an hour.
- Add bay leaves to marinades, soups, and stews to help with digestion; remove before eating, since the edges can be jagged.
- Create a decoction (see Chapter 2 for instructions) and pour into a warm bath; this helps to relieve minor aches and pains in muscles and joints. This is a perfect soak if you've overdone the gardening during the day while tending to your formidable herb collection.

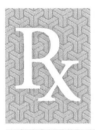

MEDICINE CABINET

Bay leaves have been used to treat a range of maladies, from digestive issues to skin problems. Herbalists often use a bay leaf poultice to help wounds heal faster, and a 2006 study found that rats treated with bay leaf extract experienced accelerated wound healing. Other studies have focused on the herb's antimicrobial properties.

Promising treatment for diabetes and cardiovascular diseases

Participants who received a small amount of ground bay leaf every day for 30 days experienced a decrease in blood glucose, cholesterol, and triglycerides. Researchers noted that consumption of bay leaves "decreases risk factors for diabetes and cardiovascular diseases and suggests that bay leaves may be beneficial for people with type 2 diabetes."[1]

Potential for inhibiting tumor growth

Researchers looked at cultivated and wild laurel samples, including bay leaves, and found evidence that the properties contained within the plants worked to inhibit certain tumor cell growth. They also noted that each laurel extract had different bioactive properties, which means that some may be more effective against bacteria, fungi, or tumors than others.[2]

1. Khan, A., et al. "Bay Leaves Improve Glucose and Lipid Profile of People with Type 2 Diabetes," *Journal of Clinical Biochemistry and Nutrition.* Jan 2009; 44(1): 52-56. http://www.ncbi.nlm.nih.gov/pmc/articles/PMC2613499/

2. Dias, M., et al. "Two-Dimensional PCA Highlights the Differentiated Antitumor and Antimicrobial Activity of Methanolic and Aqueous Extracts of *Laurus nobilis* L. from Different Origins," *BioMed Research International.* vol. 2014, article ID 520464. http://www.hindawi.com/journals/bmri/2014/520464/

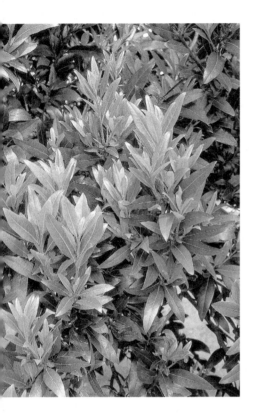

Bay laurels can be ornamental as well as useful.

PLANT·GROW·HARVEST·USE

Bay leaves are plucked from a hardy tree called a bay laurel, which can reach up to 60 feet in its native Mediterranean landscape, but tend to be much smaller and more manageable, especially if being grown indoors as a houseplant. The bay laurel does very well in a container, and its glossy, thick leaves make it a nice ornamental for walkways, or tucked into the corner of a room inside. If planting outdoors, the tree does best in Zones 8 to 11 (see USDA Hardiness Zones map on pages 22 to 23), since it prefers full sun and warmer weather.

VARIETIES Bay laurel can also be known as sweet bay or Grecian bay, and when choosing from a nursery, be sure to check the name carefully. There are a few plants that have "laurel" in their name that are potentially toxic. Steer away from common laurel, cherry laurel, poet's laurel, mountain laurel, or English laurel—these are beautiful ornamentals and resemble *Laurus nobilis* but should *never* be eaten. In terms of specific varieties, these rarely appear in seed descriptions or on transplants, and most nurseries or seed purveyors simply mark the plant as "bay laurel."

PLANT Bay laurel is so well-suited to indoor growing that it's usually best to put the shrub-like tree in a large container, which can be placed outside in warm months. The trees do best with soil that drains well, so augment potting soil with an amendment that will allow the water to flow through—one of the best choices is "cactus mix," designed to improve drainage. Blend half of that mix with half potting soil.

If growing outside, pick a spot with full sunshine and soil that *drains well.* Compacted soil will result in slow growth, or even no growth at all, so if the soil of your chosen laurel spot seems dense, loosen up the area with a pitchfork or other cultivating tool. Also, keep in mind that the plant will likely last for decades if kept healthy, so pick a spot where it can thrive for the long-term.

Instead of seeding, the best option is to buy an already-established containerized bay laurel from a greenhouse or nursery. I promise, this isn't cheating; laurels can be fussy to grow from seed, so getting a strong start with one that's mature and healthy is a nice shortcut toward an earlier harvest. The plant is so notoriously difficult to grow in its early stages that some seed companies only ship bay laurel as a plant.

GROW Once established, bay laurel requires minimal care, beyond staying on top of its watering needs. The tree doesn't do well with particularly dry or especially wet soil, so if there have been heavy rains lately, let the soil dry out for a few days before watering again.

Like all plants, a laurel also needs some amount of airflow, so if growing inside, open nearby windows to create a cross-breeze, or place a small oscillating fan in the room during warmer days.

In spring and summer, fertilize around the tree's base with an all-purpose fertilizer or some compost.

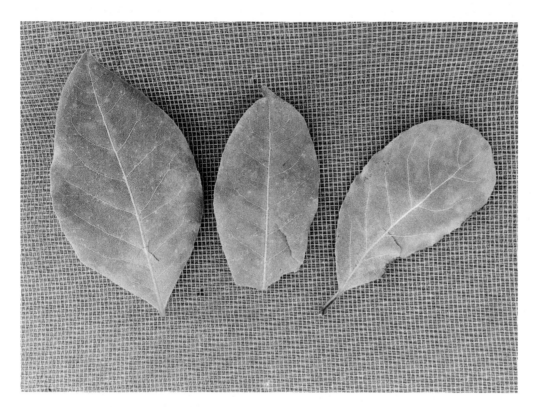

Bay leaves set out for drying usually change from green to brownish.

per 100 g (3.5 oz)

Bay leaf is rich in vitamin A, vitamin C, calcium, and potassium.

Energy	313 kcal
Carbohydrates	74.97 g
Dietary fiber	26.3 g
Fat	8.36 g
Protein	7.61 g
Water	5.44 g
Vitamin A	309 µg
Thiamine	0.009 µg
Riboflavin	0.421 mg
Niacin	2.005 mg
Vitamin B$_6$	1.740 µg
Folate	180 µg
Choline	0 mg
Vitamin C	46.5 mg
Vitamin B$_{12}$	0 mg
Vitamin K	0 µg
Calcium	834 mg
Iron	43 mg
Magnesium	120 mg
Manganese	0 mg
Phosphorus	113 mg
Potassium	529 mg
Sodium	23 mg
Zinc	3.7 mg

Source: USDA Nutrient Database

HARVEST & STORE Bay leaves can be harvested anytime of year, which is nice when it's the middle of winter and you've got a soup planned or you've got a nagging headache. The leaves tend to be more flavorful in the summer, but still retain plenty of delicious taste in other seasons. To harvest, simply pluck the leaves from the tree. Yes, it's just that easy.

If you're not going to use the leaves immediately, you can dry them with a dehydrator, but I usually just lay them out on a cooling rack—the type used to provide airflow for just-baked breads and cookies—and forget about them for a week or two. Once dried, they'll stay potent for up to a year, but they lose their flavor rapidly after that point.

Keep in mind that dried leaves don't have some of the bitter-tasting compounds that exist in fresh leaves; this is beneficial if you don't like the taste of fresh leaves, but some of the digestive healing properties that come with ingesting the herb in its bitter (fresh) form will be lost.

For cooking, simply use the entire dried or fresh leaf to add to dishes, or bundle together with sage and other herbs to make a bouquet garni. Be sure to remove the bay leaf before eating, because its brittle texture can potentially scratch your throat.

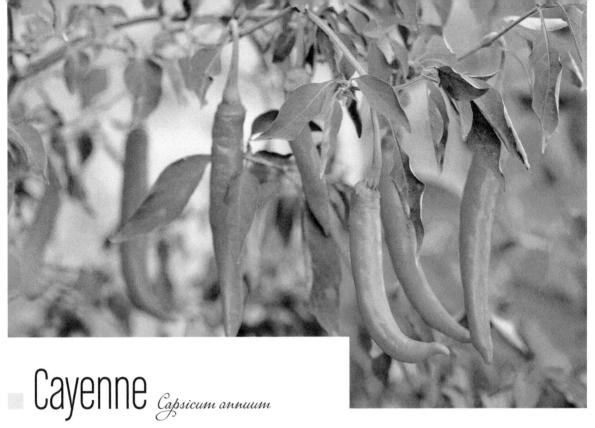

Cayenne *Capsicum annuum*

Named for the city of Cayenne in French Guiana, the cayenne pepper is also known as bird pepper, Guinea spice, and cow-horn pepper. Some estimates put pepper cultivation between 5200 and 3400 BCE, making them among the oldest cultivated plants in the world. Cayenne was introduced into the Americas in the 1500s, and has been used for culinary and medicinal purposes ever since. Today, cayenne is still recognized for its range of uses. Personally, I use the spice as an anti-cold remedy in the winter, by combining a teaspoon with 3 ounces of warm water, a little honey, and some crushed garlic. Taking this "shot" a few times a day whenever I feel cold symptoms coming on balances out my system within twenty-four hours.

Capsaicin works to alleviate pain by acting as a counter-irritant; the pain signals from the original condition like muscle aches or nerve pain become blocked. When eaten, cayenne stimulates stomach secretions, an action that helps to soothe the digestive tract.

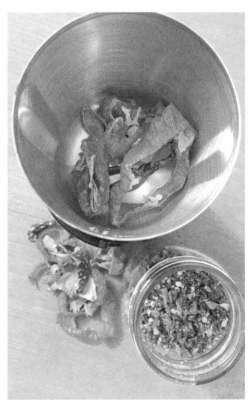

Dried peppers in a spice grinder.

Here are a few ideas for your Rx/medicinal preparations:

- Create a remedy for a sore throat by mixing ½ teaspoon dried cayenne powder (less if you're sensitive to the heat), 2 tablespoons salt, and 1 tablespoon of honey into 2 cups of water. Gently simmer the mixture for about fifteen minutes, allow it to cool until it's just warm, and gargle with ½ cup at a time.
- Address sinus congestion by putting a dash of cayenne pepper into warm water or tea and drinking it.
- For general digestion help, cook with the peppers by adding them to dishes; you can adjust heat levels by leaving out the seeds entirely, or adding some into the dish.

PLANT·GROW·HARVEST·USE

Cayenne peppers are long, red, and are ideal for drying since they tend to have thinner skins than some other types of hot peppers. Although the time from seeding to harvest can be a few months, it's worth the wait once you see the plants loaded with so many peppers it seems like it'll collapse under the weight.

VARIETIES There are hundreds of hot pepper varieties, and pepper enthusiasts are developing new ones all the time—usually to increase the heat level. Cayenne still remains one of the most popular and dependable types, with some nice varieties within the category:

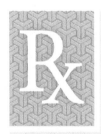
The active ingredient in cayenne peppers is capsaicin, which is what gives the peppers their heat, and causes that lovely burning sensation in the throat when you eat them. When used externally, capsaicin acts as a natural pain reliever, and has been utilized to address joint pain, headaches, and nerve pain.

Effective for pruritus ani

Itching around the anal area is both embarrassing and very common, as well as difficult to treat. But researchers have found that capsaicin ointment offered relief, leading them to conclude that "capsaicin is a new, safe, and highly effective treatment for severe intractable idiopathic pruritus ani."[1]

Aids in chronic pain

With pain caused by nerve damage, capsaicin can generate higher levels of pain relief, as well as show improvements in sleep, daytime fatigue, depression, and quality of life. High-concentration topical capsaicin is therefore similar to other therapies for chronic pain, researchers noted.[2]

1. Lysy, J., et al. "Topical capsaicin—a novel and effective treatment for idiopathic intractable pruritus ani: a randomized, placebo controlled, crossover study." Gut Sep 2003; 52(9): 1323-1326. http://www.ncbi.nlm.nih.gov/pubmed/12912865
2. Derry, S., et al. "Topical capsaicin (high concentration) for chronic neuropathic pain in adults," Cochrane Database Syst Rev. 2013; 2:CD007393. http://www.ncbi.nlm.nih.gov/pubmed/23450576

- **Joe's Long Cayenne:** these slender peppers are perfect for drying, and the thin size makes them look nice hanging in a kitchen too.
- **Cheyenne:** sweeter than many cayenne varieties, this one has thicker walls, so they don't dry as quickly as others, but they're better for cooking.
- **Red Flame:** boasts a sweet-hot taste, and the plants are very productive, to the point where you'll see more peppers than leaves when they're mature.

PLANT With cayenne, and other hot peppers, either buy already-established plants from a nursery or start the seeds indoors. Although you can go the traditional route with seed starting (place seed in soil, cover, give water, sun, and fussy attention), there's a way to speed germination time, which is especially helpful if you're getting started with peppers later in the season than you'd planned.

To kick off germination, get more moisture in the seeds by first dampening two paper towels and placing the seeds in a single layer across one of them, putting the other dampened paper towel on top. Seal the seeds and paper towels into a plastic bag (ziptop is great), or in a plastic container with a lid. Keep the bag or container in a warm area such as a kitchen, or near (but not on) a heater. Check the seeds after a few days; they should seem puffy, or even starting to sprout. Now you get to plant.

Sow each seed about ½ inch deep in a small pot that has holes for drainage, using an indoor soil mix that has a bit of fertilization in it, like worm castings or compost. Even if you're going to grow the peppers indoors—which is completely doable, if you've got some nice sunlight—choose a pot that's an appropriate size, around 3 inches deep, since that will help the start's roots stay warm and cozy. Cover the pot with plastic wrap to help retain moisture and temperature. Take off the wrap when you start to see germination.

Maturing peppers will turn from green to their final color over a matter of weeks.

Warmth is crucial when germinating the seeds and getting them started, so if your house is on the colder side, like under 65 degrees Fahrenheit, consider investing in a germination mat. These look like little heating pads, but they don't get hot to that degree. Instead, they warm the seed pots from underneath, creating a nice environment for a growing pepper and other starts.

Once the cayenne is germinated, which should be about two to four weeks after planting, keep it going with warmth and thorough watering. Peppers thrive with regular watering, and you should mist or water when the soil is just beginning to look dry. When the plant is about 6 to 8 inches tall, you can transfer to a larger pot for indoor growing, or plant outside in your garden, making sure to choose a spot with full sun and well-draining soil. Peppers appreciate slightly acidic soil, so work in compost or another natural fertilizer before planting, which will increase acidity. Plant about 2 feet apart.

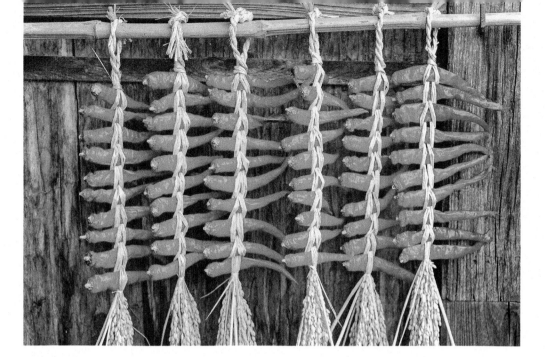

You can dry peppers by hanging them, for better air circulation.

GROW As pepper plants are adjusting to their new garden home, weed around them regularly, and consider mulching around the base, to retain moisture in the soil. Make sure to water often, since peppers tend to do best when they're properly hydrated.

If you're growing the peppers indoors, place the pot outside when it's sunny and over 60 degrees Fahrenheit, since the airflow helps the plant to get stronger. If that's not an option, just place in a sunny spot near a window that can open. Peppers need at least eight hours of sunlight every day, and they thrive with warm temperatures.

Whether indoors or outside, the peppers should begin to produce after about two to three months, depending on variety. This will feel like a very long time, I know. But once those peppers start popping, they should become abundant before long.

HARVEST & STORE Peppers start out green, and then change gradually to their final color in a process that's stunning to watch. They're ready to pick when they feel softened—occasionally "pinch" the peppers are they're growing to get a feel for when the peppers start to mature.

Once you pick them, either use them fresh or dry them. For the latter, thread a string through the stems and hang them in a dry, warm area, or use a food dehydrator. If going that route, just be sure to put the dehydrator in a *well-ventilated space;* when I first started drying peppers, I used the machine in my kitchen and loaded it up with hot peppers. After about an hour, it felt like I was trying to make homemade mace—everyone was coughing and rubbing their eyes—so the dehydrator got banished to the porch.

When the peppers are dried, they store very well in a glass jar, or you can use them immediately by crushing them in a spice grinder or coffee grinder. The resulting mix will be moist, so before storing the crushed pepper, spread the mixture evenly out on a clean cloth or paper towel and let it dry some more. Store the mix in a glass container with a tight-sealing lid.

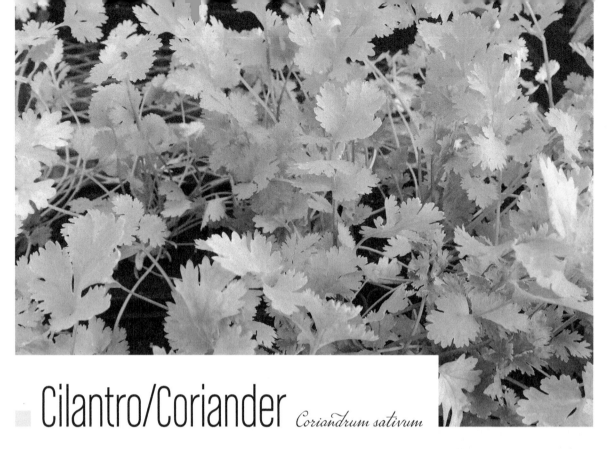

Cilantro/Coriander *Coriandrum sativum*

Also known as coriander, Chinese parsley, or dhania, cilantro seeds were found in the tomb of Tutankhamen, and the herb has been cultivated in Greece since at least the second millennium BCE. Some evidence has suggested it was once used to make perfume, but it's always been a beloved flavoring. Brought to the British colonies in North America in the 17th century, cilantro was one of the first spices cultivated in the United States by those early settlers. Despite its rich history, cilantro has a way of dividing people into lovers or haters, but if you're on the fence, a glimpse at the herb's strong anti-inflammation effects might make cilantro taste more delicious to you.

Cilantro contains antioxidants, which are incredibly helpful for preventing illness and addressing issues like inflammation. The best herbal preparation for cilantro I've found is simply eating it, but there are other methods that can come in handy if you don't like the taste.

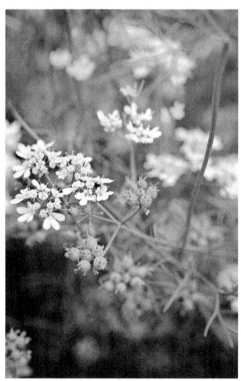

Flowering coriander with seeds.

Here are a few ideas for your Rx/medicinal preparations:

- For indigestion, dry some cilantro leaves and steep them in hot water for a tea; the flavor will be different from the fresh leaves, and you can add honey if you need a sweetener.
- Make a poultice by mashing fresh leaves into a paste with a mortar and pestle or in a blender (with a few drops of water), then spreading that over a clean cloth, which you put over the skin. Leave on for about fifteen to twenty minutes. This is particularly effective for arthritis pain.
- To take advantage of cilantro's antiviral and antifungal properties on minor wounds, sprinkle some dried, crushed cilantro on the scrape or wound, allow to sit for a few minutes, then wash the wound, dry it, and bandage.

PLANT·GROW·HARVEST·USE

Cheery and abundant (sometimes *too* abundant for some gardeners), cilantro germinates quickly, can be sown throughout spring and summer, and does well with indoor growing. The herb's abundant leaves and edible stems dry very well, and when it's bolted (going to seed, an indication that it's done with its growing season), the result is pretty white flowers that can look nice along a landscaped path.

VARIETIES Unlike some herbs, cilantro doesn't have a huge range of varieties, and most will look very similar, with flat, toothed leaves. But there are some considerations, like bolting, that can steer your choice of variety. All of these have medicinal properties, and are fairly easy to grow:

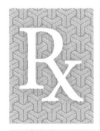

MEDICINE CABINET

All parts of a cilantro plant are edible, and people tend to favor the fresh leaves and dried seeds for cooking. But in terms of medicinal properties, even the roots and stems can be used for both culinary and wellness purposes.

Antibacterial action

Researchers found that certain properties of fresh coriander leaves were found to possess bactericidal activity against *Salmonella choleraesuis*, a food-borne bacterium.[1]

Treatment for type 2 diabetes

A study on mice found that coriander extract created insulin-like activity, and assisted the mice in releasing insulin within their own systems. Researchers noted that this was promising for potential type 2 diabetes treatments.[2]

1. Kubo, I., et al. "Antibacterial Activity of Coriander Volatile Compounds Against Salmonella choleraesuis." J. Agric. Food Chem. 2004; 52(11): 3329-3332. http://pubs.acs.org/doi/abs/10.1021/jf0354186
2. Eidi, M., et al. "Effect of coriander seed ethanol extract on insulin release from pancreatic beta cells in streptozotocin-induced diabetic rats." *Phytotherapy Research* 2009; 23(3): 404-6. http://onlinelibrary.wiley.com/resolve/doi?DOI=10.1002/ptr.2642

CHECKLIST

Sun: Four to six hours per day

Shade: Partial sun; aim for shady spot during hottest part of the day

Soil: Well-drained, loosened soil

Fertilizer: Usually not necessary, the plant can do well with minimal intervention and inputs

Pests: Tend to be minimal

Water: Regularly, depending on soil dryness

Grow Indoors? Yes, but it's fussy

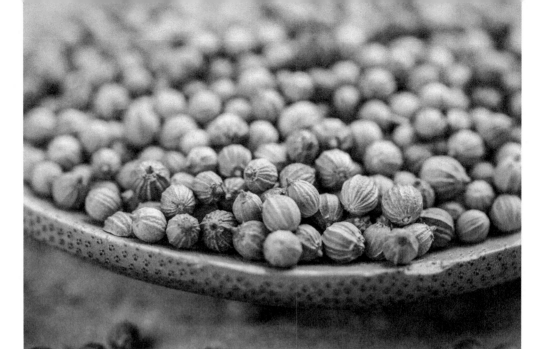

Coriander seeds are ideal for grinding.

- **Calypso:** Sometimes a range of weather conditions can cause cilantro to bolt early, limiting harvest. This variety has been cultivated as very slow to bolt, and offers a high yield of leaves.
- **Santo:** A very popular choice among growers, and if you're getting cilantro from the grocery store, it's likely that you're buying Santo. The variety is easy to grow, and tolerates cooler conditions.
- **Santo Monogerm:** Cilantro seeds are actually fruits that contain more than one seed within them, which is why the plants get so thick and bushy. If you're looking for more precise planting, choose this variety of individual seeds.
- **Caribe:** Compared to Santo, this variety has thinner stems and better bolt tolerance, and it's favored by greenhouse growers and indoor gardeners.

PLANT Cilantro does well with direct seeding into a garden space, but can be easily transplanted if you purchase a start from a nursery. Ideally, plant in the spring since this herb prefers cooler temperatures, or plant in fall if you're in warmer climates like Zones 8 to 10.

Choose a spot where the herb can stretch out and become abundant; but if you're working with smaller garden spaces, it may be advisable to plant cilantro in a container to keep it controlled. Most important, find an area that gets early morning or late afternoon sun, but is shaded during the hottest part of the day, since cilantro appreciates a break from the heat. This herb can grow in full sun, and we do that all the time on our farm, but we've noticed that the growing season is shorter since heat makes cilantro bolt faster.

Either way, you can boost germination by first soaking cilantro seeds in water for 24 to 48 hours. This allows water to get into the seed and gives it a head-start on growing. Soaking can also increase the chance of germination for older seeds. If you've had problems growing cilantro in the past through direct seeding into the garden, consider starting the plants indoors and transplanting when the starts are about 2 inches tall.

If you're eager to have plenty of cilantro, plant new seeds indoors or into the garden about every six weeks so you can replace the bolted plants with new ones.

GROW Like many herbs, cilantro does well with frequent harvesting, which encourages more growth, especially during the summer. When finished with the initial harvest season, just let it flower so that it can keep going strong and reseed, extending its next growing season, especially in the fall when cooler weather begins.

In terms of maintenance, cilantro is an easygoing addition to the herb mix, and doesn't require much care beyond occasional watering. If the plant seems to be subject to insects like aphids, either buy an organic insecticidal soap or make your own by mixing a mild liquid soap (as unscented and as preservative-free as possible) with water and spraying on the leaves.

HARVEST & STORE Since regular harvesting increases the lifespan of a cilantro plant, plan on clipping off growth fairly consistently. Rather than looking for new growth, as you would on many other types of herbs, you can harvest cilantro by just lopping off the top third of the plant; the new leaves will come from what's left behind. Ideally, you should be harvesting about once a week, but it could be more often if the cilantro is hearty.

To store, dry the leaves and stems by placing on a clean mesh surface, such as cheesecloth or a plastic screen, or tie them in small bundles and hang them in your kitchen or other area that receives adequate airflow.

Fresh cilantro also freezes beautifully—often, I throw a bunch in a food processor with a dash of lemon juice and a small amount of olive oil and pulse until it's a paste. Then, I put that into silicon ice cube trays and freeze overnight, popping them out in the morning into freezer bags. That way, I can either cook with the herb in the winter, or defrost a small amount to put into a poultice for scrapes or pain.

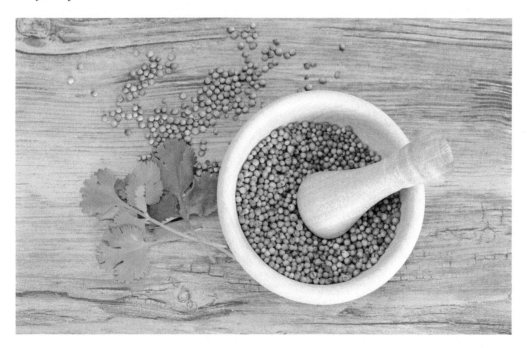

NUTRITIONAL VALUE OF CILANTRO

per 100 g (3.5 oz)

Cilantro is rich in potassium, vitamin A, vitamin K, and vitamin C.

Energy	23 kcal
Carbohydrates	3.67 g
Dietary fiber	2.8 g
Fat	0.52 g
Protein	2.13 g
Water	92.21 g
Vitamin A	337 µg
Thiamine	0.067 µg
Riboflavin	0.162 mg
Niacin	1.114 mg
Vitamin B_6	0.149 µg
Folate	62 µg
Choline	0 mg
Vitamin C	27 mg
Vitamin E	2.50 mg
Vitamin K	310.0 µg
Calcium	67 mg
Iron	1.77 mg
Magnesium	26 mg
Manganese	0 mg
Phosphorus	48 mg
Potassium	521 mg
Sodium	46 mg
Zinc	0.50 mg

Source: USDA Nutrient Database

Fresh cilantro and ground coriander seeds combine nicely for medicinal preparations.

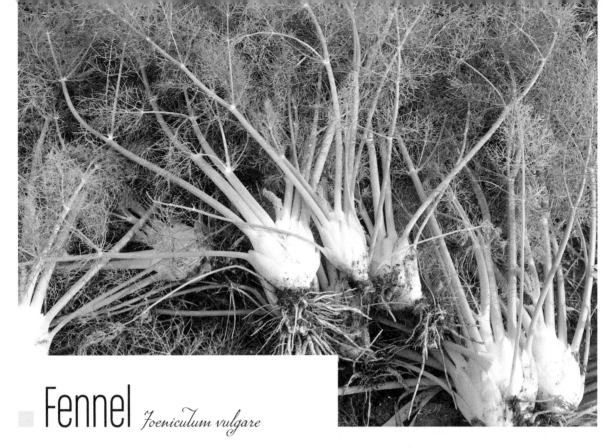

Fennel *Foeniculum vulgare*

Looking very much like its relative, dill, fennel has a licorice scent and flavor, and boasts a wealth of culinary uses as well as medicinal properties. If you've ever been to an Indian restaurant, it's likely you've seen a small bowl of fennel seeds (sometimes mixed with cardamom and anise seeds) near the register—that's because this herb is used to freshen breath and aid digestion, acting on the smooth muscles of the stomach and intestines, as well as respiratory passages. Hint: that means take a few seeds the next time, and eat them on the way to your car. Because you can use fennel bulbs, fronds, and seeds, they make a great addition to any backyard garden, giving you plenty to use for cooking as well as medicinal remedies.

Fennel is best known for its ability to soothe a bumpy digestive system, and research has noted positive effects on the

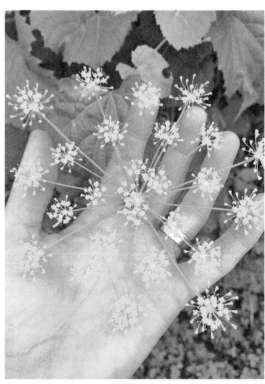

Fennel seeds are easily harvested.

liver. Since you can use all parts of the plant, from roots to seeds, it makes a good all-around choice as a tonic.

Here are a few ideas for your Rx/medicinal preparations:

- Chew on fennel seeds to freshen breath and aid in digestion. They're safe to swallow too; just be sure to chew thoroughly.
- In the fall, dig up some roots, clean thoroughly, and make a decoction by simmering the roots for about an hour, then straining through cheesecloth. Drink the strained liquid as a general tonic, or a detoxifier for the liver.
- For irritated skin on the face, place fresh fennel leaves in a bowl and pour in boiling water; lean over the bowl with your head partially covered with a towel for a cleansing steam inhalation.

PLANT·GROW·HARVEST·USE

There are actually two categories of fennel: leaf and bulb. Both offer similar culinary and medicinal uses and result in edible seeds, stems, and leaves, but true to their names, the leaf fennel is mainly feathery foliage with some tender stems, whereas the bulb fennel has a rounded base just above the roots and is considered more of a vegetable than an herb. On our farm, we've grown both types and used them

CHECKLIST

Sun: Six to ten hours per day

Shade: Full sun

Soil: Well-drained, loosened, fertile soil

Fertilizer: Minimal

Pests: Tend to be minimal

Water: Regularly; requires adequate irrigation for high yields

Grow Indoors? No

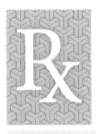

MEDICINE CABINET

Found throughout the world, fennel has a pleasant, anise flavor and is used in both its vegetable and seed form. The herb is used for various digestive problems, and also works well for respiratory tract issues like bronchitis and coughs.

Helpful for osteoporosis

A major bone disorder in elderly woman, osteoporosis has often been treated with estrogen in hormone replacement therapy. However, that treatment is usually accompanied by effects like increased susceptibility to breast and ovarian cancers. Researchers noted that the situation is increasing demand for replacement with plant phytoestrogens, and that fennel shows promise for osteoprotective effects.[1]

Promising for colic

In a trial of 125 infants with colic, about 40 percent of infants receiving fennel showed relief of symptoms, compared with only 14 percent of those in the placebo group. Researchers noted that the results are promising and that more study should be done to confirm fennel's efficacy for treatment.[2]

1. Mahmoudi, Z. "Effects of Foeniculum vulgare ethanol extract on osteogenesis in human mecenchymal stem cells," *Avicenna J Phytomed* 2013 Spring;3(2):135–42. http://www.ncbi.nlm.nih.gov/pubmed/25050267

2. http://www.med.nyu.edu/content?ChunkIID=108303#ref1

mainly for cooking, since we often use up our herbs before letting them go to seed. But several farmer friends have noted that allowing the fennel to go to seed results in some delicious teas.

VARIETIES The variety of fennel you choose will most likely depend on your garden space and your interest in eating the bulbs. Although I find the bulbs unbelievably delicious, their anise flavor isn't for everyone. If you're interested just in teas, seeds, and using the fronds, leaf fennel may be a better choice since the flavor isn't as strong. Either way, there are plenty of nice options:

- **Orion:** a bulb fennel that produces large, thick rounded bulbs and solid stems that can be used like a licorice-infused celery.
- **Zefa Fino:** Most fennel requires planting in the spring to prevent bolting, but this bulb variety was bred to be more bolt resistant, so you can plant it in the summer.
- **Bronze:** if you're looking for an ornamental plant as well as a medicinal one, this variety works well since it has a beautiful reddish gold color and tends to be shorter than bulb fennel. The leaves also make a lovely addition when sprinkled on top of dishes, thanks to its distinctive color.
- **Grosfruchtiger:** a green leaf fennel, this variety has vigorous leaf production and tends to be sweeter tasting than other fennels, making it nice for a lighter, sweeter tea.

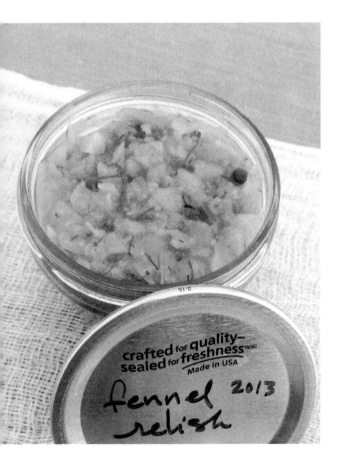

Fennel relish is simple to make. I get my recipe from the *Ball Complete Book of Home Preserving*.

PLANT Fennel can be planted into a garden as a transplant, but most often, it's directly seeded into a garden space in the late spring. For those in Zones 5 to 10, congratulations! Fennel is a perennial that can survive your winters and come back in the spring. But for those of us living in the refrigerator section of the US, you'll have to consider the plant an annual, reseeding or replanting each year.

Before planting, loosen up the soil and add some compost (non-manure kind, so you're not boosting the nitrogen too high). Fennel seeds only need a very light covering of soil, so plant close to the surface, about 10 inches apart for leaf fennel and 18 inches apart for bulb fennel, and sprinkle with soil. Be sure to water thoroughly—but gently, given the seeds' position—as the seeds start to establish.

One important, quirky note: if you also have dill growing in your garden, separate that herb from the fennel. Put them on opposite sides of a garden, if possible. That's because fennel and dill will cross-pollinate if given the chance, and although we all appreciate a story of forbidden love, you'll end up with strange-tasting seeds if you're using those for teas and salads.

GROW Fennel doesn't require much care beyond occasional watering, making it an easy addition to a garden. If you find

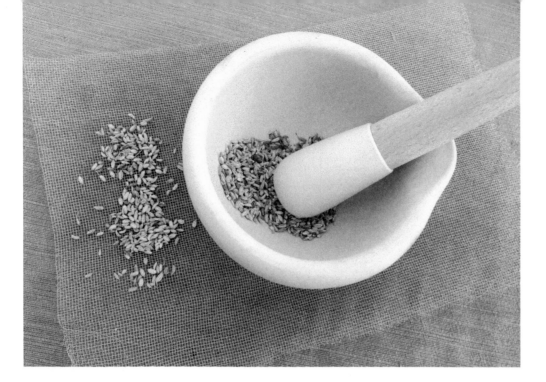

Crushing seeds with a mortar and pestle.

NUTRITIONAL VALUE OF FENNEL SEED

per 100 g (3.5 oz)

Fennel seed is rich in potassium, magnesium, calcium, vitamin C, and phosphorus.

Energy	345 kcal
Carbohydrates	52.29 g
Dietary fiber	39.8 g
Fat	14.87 g
Protein	15.8 g
Water	8.81 g
Vitamin A	7 µg
Thiamine	0.408 µg
Riboflavin	0.353 mg
Niacin	6.050 mg
Vitamin B$_6$	0.470 µg
Folate	0 µg
Choline	0 mg
Vitamin C	21.0 mg
Vitamin E	0 mg
Vitamin K	0 µg
Calcium	1196 mg
Iron	18.54 mg
Magnesium	385 mg
Manganese	0 mg
Phosphorus	487 mg
Potassium	1694 mg
Sodium	88 mg
Zinc	3.70 mg

Source: USDA Nutrient Database

that it's struggling in any way, consider misting around the roots with a mixture of water and fish emulsion (available at any garden store). In general, we call this blend "the magic juice" because it's helpful for just about any issue we're seeing, from yellowing leaves to drooping tomatoes.

HARVEST & STORE Picking fennel is just as easy as maintaining it in a garden. Simply cut off the stems of leaf fennel as you need them, taking care to leave the small, compact new growth alone. These new growth leaves are easy to spot since they're very compact and usually brightly colored.

For bulb fennel, you can harvest the stems with their leafy fronds, but most likely, you'll be pulling up the whole bulb once it reaches adequate size, which depends on the variety. Some bulbs are round, like tennis balls, while others are flat, like side plates. Either way, grasp the bulb on each side, close to the ground, and pull. The whole bulb should come up with roots.

Then, you can dry the fronds for tea and put the bulb in the fridge for eating. If you're looking to use the seeds, harvest those in the fall after the flowers have turned brown—leave the seeds to dry on the plant rather than collecting them and drying them on a screen. The seeds should come off the plant very easily, so put some kind of container underneath and brush the seeds off. Put the seeds in an airtight, glass jar and they should keep for at least six months; be sure to check them after the first week or so to make sure they're dried enough and are not developing mold.

Fennel seeds are delicious, but if you have a fennel bulb and the feathery fronds, there's a wealth of culinary possibilities. Usually, I coarsely chop the bulb, coat with olive oil, and grill for five minutes per side—the result is a caramelized, sumptuous side dish that goes well with the other grill-worthy fennel dish: salmon drizzled with butter, tucked into aluminum foil, and chopped-up fronds layered inside. Seriously delicious.

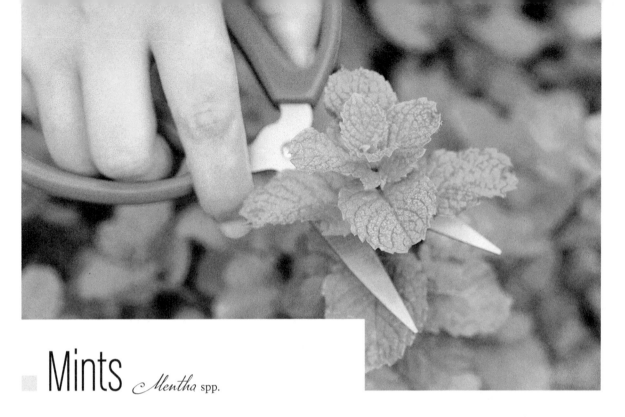

Mints *Mentha* spp.

For this section, I decided to showcase a genus of herbs rather than discuss how to plant, grow, and use one specific species, like peppermint or spearmint. Although each mint certainly has its distinctive flavors, they tend to grow under the same conditions and can be used interchangeably in medicinal and culinary preparations. Honestly, I just love them all and it's hard to pick a favorite, so I didn't. In terms of history, "mint" comes from Menthe, a nymph in Greek mythology who was turned into a ground-clinging plant by jealous Persephone. Hades softened the transition by giving her the ability to sweeten the air when her leaves were pressed, but it doesn't seem like much of a consolation. Still, that nymph sure does make a nice mint julep.

Most varieties of mint have stimulating properties, which is what makes them so ideal for digestion, and peppermint boasts additional antimicrobial and anti-spasmodic properties, making that mint particularly nice for chronic conditions like irritable bowel syndrome.

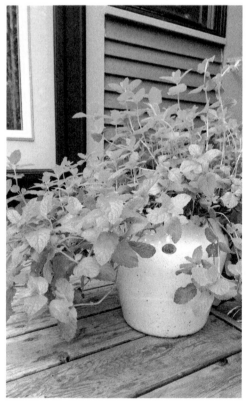

Putting mint in pots helps to keep them from becoming invasive to the rest of your garden.

Here are a few ideas for your Rx/medicinal preparations:

- Create an energy booster by first creating an infusion of 2 teaspoons of fresh peppermint leaves steeped in just-boiled water, then pouring into a warm bath.
- Dry mint leaves on a screen and make a tea that can be used to reduce indigestion. You can play around with tea strength by increasing the amount of leaves; just be sure to let it steep for only a few minutes. Any longer than that and the tea will get bitter. Start with about 2 heaping tablespoons of dried leaves to 16 ounces of very hot (not boiling) water.
- To help with digestion issues, chop fresh leaves and put on a salad, or put whole leaves into fresh water or lemonade.

PLANT·GROW·HARVEST·USE

A common refrain for gardeners is that once you have mint you'll always have mint. The leafy plant establishes quickly and spreads easily—perhaps a little too easily, in some cases. Mint can become invasive if left unchecked, and although it imparts a sweet aroma and flavor to dishes and medicinal

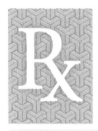

MEDICINE CABINET

Mint has been used throughout history for digestion issues and stomach problems, as well as to freshen breath, so it's no surprise that so many commercial toothpastes and antacids would feature mint flavorings.

Antimicrobial activity

An antimicrobial agent can kill microorganisms or inhibit growth, providing benefits against bad bacteria that can spread illness. Researchers noted that all extracts from *Mentha longifolia* showed different ranges of antimicrobial activities, and all showed antifungal activities against *Candida albicans,* a fungus that causes yeast issues in the body.[1]

Effective for chronic pain

The use of traditional medicine has been growing in the treatment of bladder pain syndrome, due to its high prevalence and insufficient treatment by conventional therapies, researchers noted. Researchers administered mint to register its effect as one of the more traditional herbs for pain in a patient with the syndrome. They found that in one patient with the diagnosis, there was a marked alleviation of signs and symptoms, suggesting further studies are needed.[2]

1. Bakht, J. "Report: Antimicrobial potentials of Mentha longifolia by disc diffusion method," *Pak J Pharm Sci* 2014 Jul; 27(4):939-45. http://www.ncbi.nlm.nih.gov/pubmed/25015464
2. Latifi, S.A., et al. "Complementary treatment in chronic pelvic pain syndrome: a case report study," *Iran Red Crescent Med J* 2014 Apr; 16(4):e13681. http://www.ncbi.nlm.nih.gov/pubmed/24910801

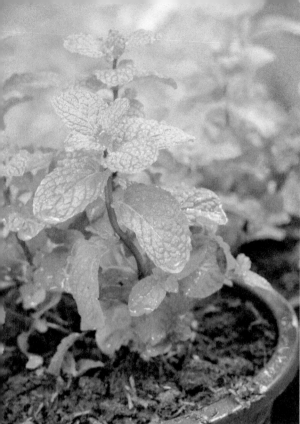

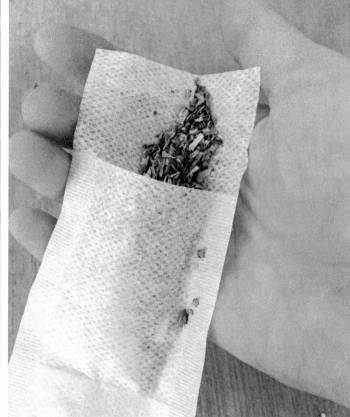

Left: Mint in smaller pots can be ideal for indoor growing.

Right: Dried mint placed in a teabag, for drinking or putting into a bath.

preparations, most people don't want to become mint growers. Because of that, it's sometimes advisable to grow mint in a container so it can be controlled, or to grow it inside, where it can be quickly harvested.

VARIETIES Once you begin to peruse seed catalogs, you'll see why I couldn't confine myself to describe just one variety of mint. There are mints that hail from Korea, the Middle East, South America, and China. Some impart a slight licorice flavor or feature edible flowers that can dried for sweet tea, while others smell like apple, or feature boosted spearmint flavor. One herb purveyor even offers a seven-mint set for those who can't decide. Here's just a sampling:

- **Arabian:** with downy leaves and light blue leaves, this variety makes a pretty ornamental as well as a solid medicinal.
- **Chinese:** used in traditional Chinese medicine to address fever, cough, sore throat, and irritated eyes, this variety has hearty leaves and a spearmint flavor.
- **Doublemint:** with rounded leaves, this spearmint variety are particularly vigorous and good for container growing.
- **Applemint:** with fuzzy leaves and an apple aroma, this variety is an excellent choice for teas, and makes a nice ornamental along walkways.
- **Mayan:** considered a rare mint (although still available for purchase at some seed companies), with cone-like flowers and very sweet taste. The leaves have a purplish tint and the plant sends out runners, meaning that it drapes beautifully over rock walls.
- **Peppermint:** a dependable variety with a familiar taste. Classic leaves, happy flavor, and dries well.

PLANT Mints are fast-growing plants that spread so quickly I've seen gardeners put them inside of a pot, and then put that pot inside of a container of other herbs or inside the ground. The herb sends out runners to claim more space, creating a lush bush that makes a good groundcover if you don't mind the expansion.

Plant in the spring—or if you live in a climate without frost, you can plant in the fall as well—by direct seeding, or by taking a cutting of an existing mint plant from a friend or neighbor.

Because mint is so popular, it's often found in nurseries, even in less-common options like chocolate mint or sweet mint. Because of that, it may be easiest to simply buy a transplant, since it will already be established and can be transferred directly to a garden space or indoor container.

When choosing a garden spot, consider using mint as a companion plant; because of its natural oils, the mint helps to deter insects from a number of vegetables, such as beets, broccoli, kale, kohlrabi, and others. Mint planted near tomatoes, cabbage, and peas reportedly improves the flavor and health of those plants.

GROW Mint tends to start blooming early, and will continue blooming from June to September. In order to keep the plant more compact, snip off the buds, and dry them for teas and other medicinal use.

To keep the plant more robust, trim off any yellowing lower leaves, and fertilize every two to three weeks by sprinkling some fertilizer around the roots. Make sure it's a fertilizer that's lower in salts (chat with your garden store about different brands and their salt content), otherwise the leaf tips will start to turn brown, and you can lightly mulch around the plant with straw or newspaper strips to help keep roots moist.

HARVEST & STORE Harvest mint leaves whenever you need them; like many other herbs, mints do best with frequent harvests. Fortunately, the leaves dry beautifully on a clean mesh screen or in the racks of an herb dehydrator. Then, you can crush them in a spice grinder and store in airtight glass jars.

When using fresh mint, the possibilities are seemingly endless, and all boast the kind of happy-digestion effects that you'd want in any dish. Tuck a few leaves into spring rolls, shred over salads, add to a pitcher of ice water, chop up finely and put into scrambled eggs, or combine with peas in a pasta dish.

Similar to other herbs, mint also freezes well. Throw a bunch in a food processor with a dash of lemon juice and a small amount of olive oil and pulse until it's a paste. Then, put that into silicon ice cube trays and freeze overnight, popping them out in the morning into freezer bags. In the winter, when the landscape is either snowy and bleak or brown and lackluster (depending on your location), take those frozen cubes and add to lemonade; strain once they melt, and you'll have a mint-infused drink that tastes like you're in the middle of summer.

NUTRITIONAL VALUE OF PEPPERMINT

per 100 g (3.5 oz)

Peppermint is rich in potassium and vitamin A.

Energy	70 kcal
Carbohydrates	14.89 g
Dietary fiber	8 g
Fat	0.94 g
Protein	3.75 g
Water	78.65 g
Vitamin A	212 µg
Thiamine	0.082 µg
Riboflavin	0.266 mg
Niacin	1.706 mg
Vitamin B$_6$	0.129 µg
Folate	114 µg
Choline	0 mg
Vitamin C	31.8 mg
Vitamin E	0 mg
Vitamin K	0 µg
Calcium	243 mg
Iron	5.08 mg
Magnesium	80 mg
Manganese	0 mg
Phosphorus	73 mg
Potassium	569 mg
Sodium	31 mg
Zinc	1.11 mg

Source: USDA Nutrient Database

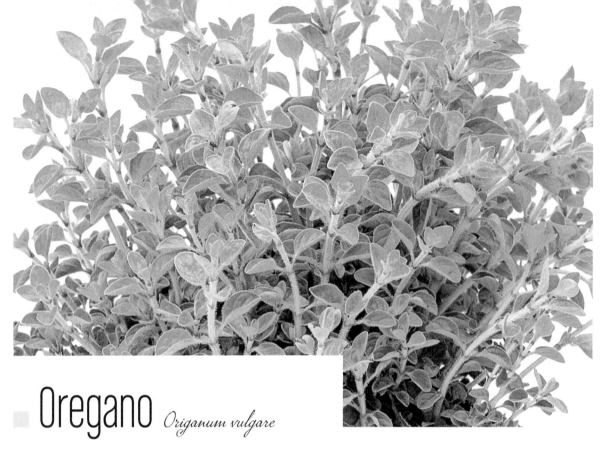

Oregano *Origanum vulgare*

Besides serving as an excellent culinary ingredient in pasta dishes and soups, oregano has quite an impressive medicinal pedigree. Hippocrates reputedly used the herb as a treatment for stomach problems and respiratory issues, as well as antiseptic uses. Oregano is still very much in vogue in Greece today as a standard treatment for sore throats. In other parts of Europe, especially Austria, the herb is used for respiratory ailments and nervous system issues. Researchers in Poland have found some immune-boosting superpowers for the herb too. When tested against seventy other herbs for immunity effects, oregano came in first place. That makes this everyday culinary choice into a real standout.

Oregano's oil-packed leaves make it a popular treatment for a range of issues, and oil of oregano can be a useful addition to any medicinal lineup. But unless you're ready to

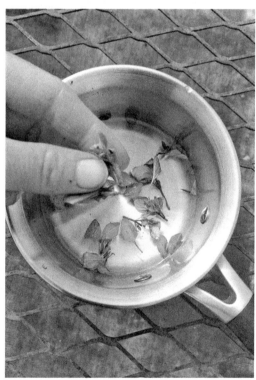

Oregano added to boiling water.

set up a still and distill your own essential oils, it's likely you'll have to find easier ways to extract the potent properties. Fortunately, there's an array of options.

Here are a few ideas for your Rx/medicinal preparations:

- Dry the leaves, and make into a tea to help treat fatigue, irritable bowel syndrome, and bacterial infections. If you're growing weary of tea (is that even possible?) you can also pack the dried leaves into empty gelatin capsules, available at many co-ops, and take in pill form.
- To help with itching and swelling on the skin, mash the fresh leaves into a paste and add a small amount of hot water to help the mixture hold together. Sprinkle in a bit of oatmeal for thickening, and to help soothe skin, and cover irritated skin. Cover with clean gauze or towel.
- Use cooled oregano tea to spray on pets, since the mixture can help kill fleas and act as an antibacterial, topical treatment that decreases itching.

PLANT·GROW·HARVEST·USE

Oregano is particularly good as a small, well-controlled part of any garden you've planted for your backyard pharmacy. Non-invasive, easy to maintain, and robust if harvested regularly, the herb does well with warm temperatures and full sun, making it a perfect summer choice for a culinary mix. The herb also does well in indoor pots, especially if you're extending the growing season. For example, oregano propagates well if you take a cutting from an existing outdoor plant and prepare it for growth

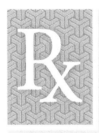

MEDICINE CABINET

Oregano is helpful for an array of maladies, from coughs and bronchitis to gastrointestinal disorders such as heartburn. It's also been recommended for urinary tract infections, parasites, allergies, and even dandruff and spider bites. Consider all *that* the next time you skip sprinkling it on your pizza.

Controls blood sugar levels

Researchers from the University of Illinois noted that oregano and rosemary contain diabetes-fighting compounds, and show promise in treating type 2 diabetes. Researchers tested four different herbs for the study, and noted that greenhouse-grown herbs contain more polyphenols and flavonoids, two beneficial compounds, when compared to equivalent commercial herbs.[1]

May protect against drug-resistant bacteria

Oregano oil may be an effective treatment against dangerous drug-resistant bacteria, a researcher noted. Two studies have shown that oil made from the herb appears to reduce infection as effectively as traditional antibiotics.[2]

1. http://zeenews.india.com/news/health/health-news/rosemary-oregano-can-fight-type-2-diabetes-study_28905.html
2. http://www.sciencedaily.com/releases/2001/10/011011065609.htm

CHECKLIST

Sun: Eight to ten hours per day

Shade: Full sun needed

Soil: Well-drained, loosened soil

Fertilizer: Usually not necessary

Pests: Tend to be minimal

Water: When the soil is dry

Grow Indoors? Yes

inside. If that's your strategy, simply cut a 4-inch section (measured from the tip of the stem/leaf toward the soil) and strip off about an inch or so of the lower leaves. Put the stem into a potting mix, such as vermiculite, and keep the mix somewhat moist as the plant establishes.

VARIETIES When people buy oregano in dried or fresh form, it's usually Greek oregano, a hearty variety with dark green leaves and a strong oregano taste and aroma. When the variety flowers, in small white blooms (similar to its relative, marjoram), it signals the end of the growth season, but they're also edible and make a nice accompaniment to salads. But don't limit yourself to a single variety—here are a few other choices:

- **Wild Zaatar:** a good medicinal variety that grows wild in Israel, Jordan, and surrounding areas; flavor contains hints of thyme and marjoram as well as oregano. Be sure to use loose, well-draining soil in order to establish.
- **Oregano Vulgare:** an Italian variety, with potent medicinal value. It does well with direct seeding compared to starting indoors as transplants. Though less flavorful than Greek oregano, it's good for attracting beneficial insects, and good companion plant for vegetables. It's especially nice as an edible ornamental, since it's taller than Greek oregano, and features lavender-pink blooms.

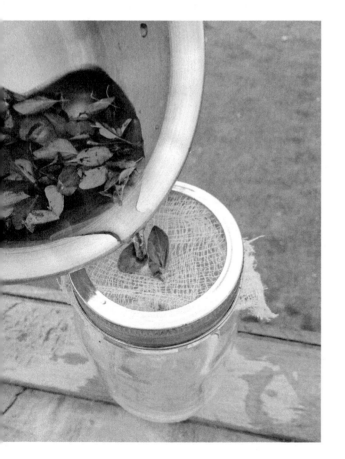

Fresh oregano leaves can be boiled and then strained through cheesecloths.

PLANT Oregano can be direct seeded into a garden, if you have just the right conditions for it, but it thrives best if it's transplanted from a start that's been nurtured indoors for at least a month. Either buy a small start from a greenhouse, or grow one yourself in a warm and cozy indoor space in early spring for planting after the last frost.

If growing outside, pick a spot with full sunshine and soil that drains well. Compacted soil will result in slow growth, or even no growth at all, so if your chosen thyme spot's soil seems dense, loosen the area with a pitchfork or other cultivating tool.

For inside growing, consider starting the seeds in a small container (about 2 inches or so) first, which will keep the roots warmer, aiding in germination. As the plant grows larger, transfer to a larger container (at least 6 inches) so the roots can establish more firmly. Whether the herb will be indoors or in a garden, put a small amount of slow-release fertilizer into the soil at the start of the season.

Sometimes oregano and other herbs can struggle if the pH of the soil is off, so in that case, test your soil to make sure it's alkaline enough for the thyme; it should be between about 6 to 8; if it's lower, boost it with a little lime sprinkled around the base of the plant.

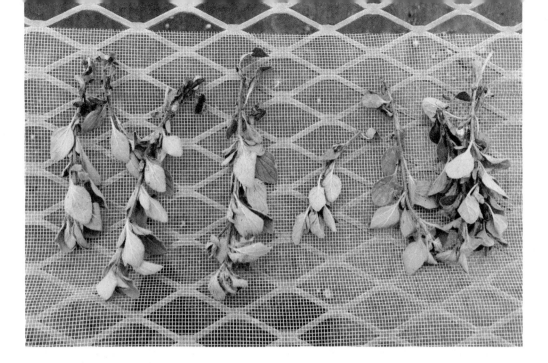

Oregano dries very well, especially on screens that allow for plenty of airflow.

GROW Like many herbs, oregano does well with frequent harvesting, which encourages more growth, especially during the summer. Allow the plant to grow to about 4 inches, then trim lightly, otherwise the plant will get dense and sometimes more woody.

Be sure to water thoroughly when it's dry, but don't water regularly. Oregano does well with minimal watering, and can be prone to root rot and insect issues if overwatered. It's much better to soak the plants when the soil feels dry, and then water less often.

After plants are about three to four years old, thin them so they have more room to grow. Oregano is self-seeding, so you should see it in your garden each spring, but if not thinned after about three years, they can get too bushy.

Finally, consider dividing the plants so some grow indoors and others in your garden. This can be done by simply digging up part of the plant, roots and all, and transplanting into a pot filled with potting soil. Oregano does very well inside, and makes a stellar addition to a small culinary kitchen garden.

HARVEST & STORE Usually, oregano is harvested as you need it, but it also freezes exceedingly well. To freeze, put in a food processor with a dash of lemon juice (to preserve color) and a small amount of olive oil and pulse until it's a paste. Then, put that mix into silicon ice cube trays (which help prevent sticking) and freeze overnight, popping them out in the morning into freezer bags. When you want to cook with the herb in the winter, just grab a little cube and throw it directly into dishes.

In the summer, I prefer to use fresh oregano for cooking and salads since I enjoy the taste, but I do dry quite a bit for winter cooking, especially near the end of the summer, when the oregano seems ready to fade. Oregano dries exceedingly well when placed together in a bundle and hung up to dry. Bundles can be stored in this form or stripped of their leaves, which are then placed in small jars for use in cooking, teas, and even small sachets that can freshen up the scent of drawers and closets.

For cooking and medicinal use, simply chop up the dried or fresh leaves and add to dishes, or store in airtight jars.

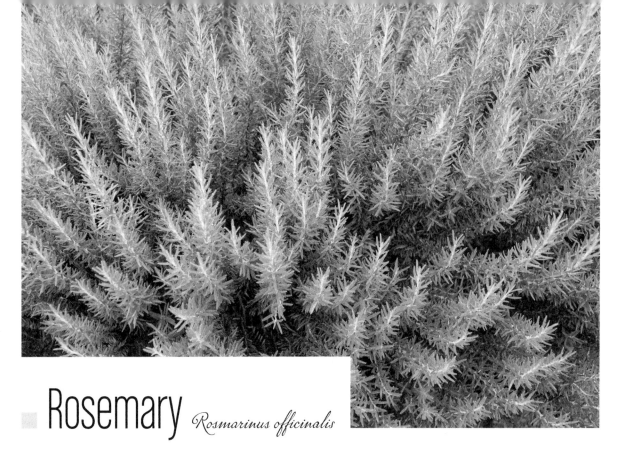

Rosemary *Rosmarinus officinalis*

Although rosemary is a common culinary spice these days, the herb has a rich history of culinary, medicinal, and even cosmetic uses. It's been used ceremonially to represent fidelity, friendship, and remembrance, particularly for important life events—brides would weave rosemary into their bouquets, and decorate pews with the herb to represent a vow of faithfulness. In Great Britain, churches would sprinkle rosemary on the floors at Christmas to remember those who'd passed during the year, and as acknowledgement of the herb's role in Christianity—reportedly, the flowers used to be white, but changed to blue when the Virgin Mary threw her cloak over a rosemary bush on the flight from Egypt. Also, rosemary reportedly lives exactly thirty-three years, the length of Christ's life. In addition to its major symbolism, the herb has been used as a hair rinse, as well as a treatment for headache, depression, and sciatia.

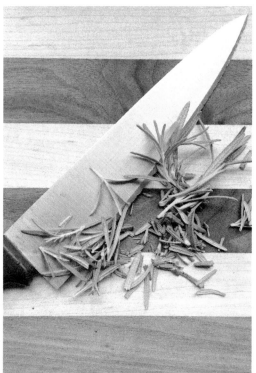

Rosemary is a great complement to many culinary dishes.

Rosemary is so plentiful that it makes a nice addition to any medicinal and culinary garden mix, particularly if it's freshly harvested. The herb is a circulatory and nervine stimulant, and has a calming effect on the digestive system.

Here are a few ideas for your Rx/medicinal preparations:

- To calm nerves or stimulate the appetite, create an infusion by pouring a cup of boiling water over a couple teaspoons of the dried herb and leaving in a covered container for about fifteen minutes. Drink up to three times per day, but don't take for more than a couple days consecutively.

- As a way to help digestion, use fresh rosemary in a mix used to marinate meat, combining the herb with ingredients like shallots, garlic, and parsley.

- For dandruff or dry scalp, create a few cups of a rosemary infusion from fresh leaves and rinse hair after shampooing.

PLANT·GROW·HARVEST·USE

Rosemary is a favorite in herb gardens and is especially good in container gardens because of its distinctive, woody look. The needlelike leaves can sometimes reach up to 3 feet in height, and even taller if not harvested. In my particular hardiness zone, the cooler temps cause our rosemary to seem stunted in comparison to warmer zones, where rosemary gets so robust that it sometimes makes good hedges. The plants are also tolerant of salt, unlike many other herbs, so it grows well in coastal areas.

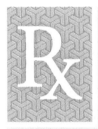

MEDICINE CABINET

Rosemary boasts an impressive number of medicinal actions and is considered a carminative, anti-spasmodic, anti-depressive, and antiseptic. Research into other actions is showing promising results for conditions that range from cancer prevention to diabetes control.

Controls blood sugar levels

Researchers from the University of Illinois noted that oregano and rosemary contain diabetes-fighting compounds, and show promise in treating type 2 diabetes. Researchers tested four different herbs for the study, and noted that greenhouse-grown herbs contain more polyphenols and flavonoids, two beneficial compounds, when compared to equivalent commercial herbs.[1]

Antioxidant and anti-tumor properties

Rosemary leaves have potent antioxidant activity, researchers noted, and the herb also inhibits skin, colon, and mammary carcinogensis, which mean that it shows promise as a treatment for preventing tumors from forming.[2]

1. http://zeenews.india.com/news/health/health-news/rosemary-oregano-can-fight-type-2-diabetes-study_28905.html

2. Chi-Tang, H., et al. "Antioxidative and Antitumorigenic Properties of Rosemary," *Functional Foods for Disease Prevention* 1998; Chapter 15, pp. 153-161. http://pubs.acs.org/doi/pdf/10.1021/bk-1998-0702.ch015

Rosemary also makes a nice choice for indoor growing, and can be included in a pot with other herbs like sage or basil.

VARIETIES Rosemary's distinctive aroma and taste have made it a favorite for chefs and herbalists alike. Harvesting is as easy as grasping the bottom of the stem and zipping off the pine needle-type leaves. When choosing a plant, many nurseries and seed purveyors often don't designate a specific variety, and instead just sell "rosemary," or "common rosemary," but there are some other varieties worth noting, which all boast a nice amount of medicinal clout:

- **Lockwood de Forest:** With lavender blue flowers, this variety makes an attractive border in ornamentals, and makes a good choice for container gardening.
- **Prostrate Rosemary:** Awkwardly named, but it's strangely fitting, since this variety has more tender stems that allow the plant to fall becomingly over the edges of pots and raised beds. A nice choice for draping over a stone wall.
- **Spice Island**: Does very well in warmer climates, and is a perennial in Zones 7 to 9. Stands upright and has very strong flavor, making it a great culinary choice.
- **Gorizia:** Named for a town in Italy where it originated, this variety is particularly mildew resistant, with unusually flat, large leaves.

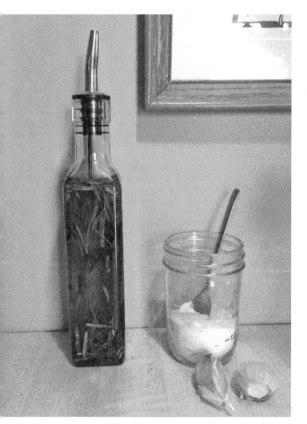

Rosemary-infused olive oil.

PLANT When considering where to plant rosemary, find a spot with full sun and well-drained, loosened soil, preferably close to your backyard entrance so you can harvest frequently.

For inside or outside growing, consider starting the seeds in a shallow container (about 2 inches or so) first, which will keep the roots warmer, aiding germination. As the plant grows larger, transfer to a larger container (at least 6 inches deep) so the roots can establish more firmly. Whether the herb will be indoors or in a garden, put a small amount of slow-release fertilizer into the soil at the start of the season.

Sometimes, rosemary and other herbs can struggle if the pH of the soil is off, so in that case, test your soil to make sure it's alkaline enough for the rosemary; it should be between 6 and 7. If it's lower, boost the pH with a little lime sprinkled around the base of the plant.

Once you've planted the rosemary, mulch around the roots to insulate in winter and keep the soil uniformly moist in the summer.

GROW Like many herbs, rosemary does well with frequent harvesting, a practice that encourages more growth, particularly during the height of the growing season. As cooler weather begins, or if you'd just like a break from harvesting, let the plant flower so

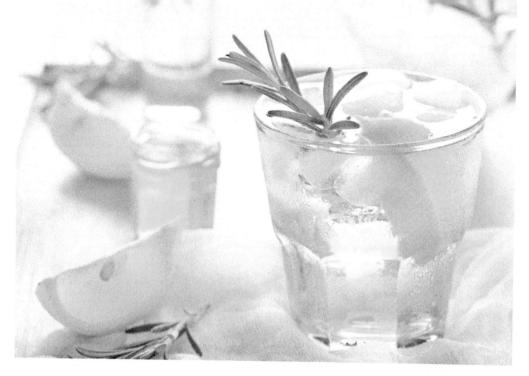

Gin with lemon and honey: now, that's medicinal.

that it can keep going strong for the next year, but be sure to trim the plant back after flowering so that it doesn't get woody with overly thick stems. Before the winter, bring the plant inside to continue growth, or prevent freeze damage by covering those plants in the garden.

In terms of maintenance, rosemary is an easygoing addition to the herb mix, and doesn't require much care beyond occasional watering. If the plant seems to be struggling, try cultivating around the base so that the soil loosens for better drainage.

Rosemary can seem to have sluggish growth when you first plant it, but the herb grows much more robust in the second season onward.

HARVEST & STORE Because rosemary has those needlelike leaves, you can harvest anytime of day, and from early summer to the end of the growing season. Harvest frequently, since this encourages more growth.

In the summer, I prefer to use fresh rosemary for remedies and medicinal preparations since the flavor and aroma are stronger. When cooking, for example, the scent of rosemary is almost intoxicating. In fact, it can be part of a drink that's literally intoxicating: a vodka rosemary lemonade fizz, which combines lemon juice, sugar, rosemary sprigs, vodka, and club soda. Hello, summer.

Rosemary also dries very well, especially when bundled and hung up to dry. You can store the bundles this way in a cool, dust-free area, or strip them of their leaves and store those. Either way, you can use the leaves for cooking, teas, and other uses.

Create a nice culinary and medicinal mix of uses through cooking. Simply chop up the dried or fresh leaves and add to dishes, use the stem as a shishkabob for meats and vegetables, or make flavored olive oil by throwing three or four sprigs into a bottle. Another favorite option here at the farm is to finely chop the fresh leaves and mix into softened butter, then to use that on salmon, bread, or sandwiches. Not only are these uses tasty, but they make the most of rosemary's calming effect on the digestion.

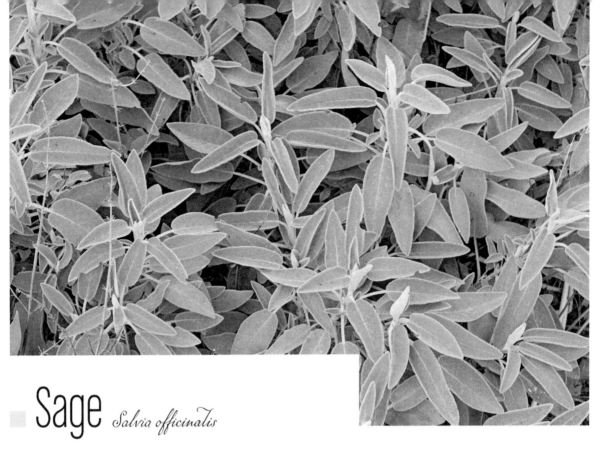

Sage *Salvia officinalis*

Sage's botanical name comes from the Latin word *salvere*, meaning to cure or to save, and the powerful little herb can be true to that definition. Although it's a favorite for culinary use, sage boasts a significant history for medicinal use, particularly in Chinese medicine, where it's used as a nerve tonic. The Greeks believed that keeping sage in a garden prevented doctor visits, and an old Chinese proverb noted that a man can't grow old with sage in his garden. Although neither of these claims seems likely to come true, it doesn't hurt to give it a try. If nothing else, the herb is divine when it comes to whipping up Italian dishes, and it dries beautifully for making into an end-of-day tonic wine or an uplifting tea anytime.

A well-known digestive, sage also works as a tonic for the nervous system to decrease anxiety and depression. As research has shown for its effects on Alzheimer's disease, sage can improve memory and increase an overall sense of well-being.

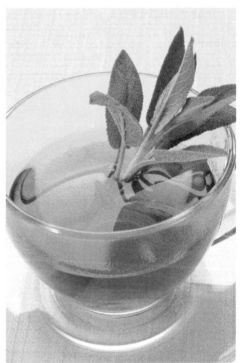

Freshly steeped sage, to be used as a gargle for a sore throat or a wellness tonic.

Here are a few ideas for your Rx/medicinal preparations:

- Prepare an infusion by steeping dried or fresh leaves in just-boiled water and allowing it to cool. Use as a gargle for a sore throat, or drink as a general wellness tonic.
- To aid digestion, put about 3 ounces of fresh leaves in a liter of dry white wine and let steep overnight. Drink a small glass before dinner.
- For helping to balance blood sugar, create a tea by drying leaves on a clean mesh screen, and then crumbling or grinding them and placing in a tea bag. Drink once per day for a few days.

PLANT·GROW·HARVEST·USE

Considered a staple of many culinary and medicinal gardens, sage is a perennial that plays well with others both in container gardens and raised beds. Although it can get bushy, the herb isn't invasive and grows easily. Its thick leaves appear almost dusty, and can be prone to picking up splashes of dirt after a rainfall. But it's generally disease resistant and simple to use for both cooking and medicinal preparations.

CHECKLIST

Sun: Six to eight hours per day

Shade: Prefers full sun

Soil: Well-drained, loosened soil; can grow in sandy soil

Fertilizer: Usually not necessary

Pests: Some, including aphids and whiteflies

Water: When soil seems dry

Grow Indoors? Yes

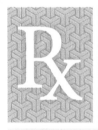

MEDICINE CABINET

With leathery, hardy leaves that dry well and work nicely in teas and other remedies, sage is an easy pick when it comes to medicinal and culinary uses. The herb has often been used for digestive issues such as bloating, stomach pain, gas, and heartburn. It's also been recommended for cold sores, menstrual problems, and gum disease.

Effective for hot flashes

Researchers undertook a trial to assess the tolerability and efficacy of fresh sage in treating hot flashes and other menopausal complaints, since sage has been used for those issues traditionally. They found that those study subjects using the sage showed significant decrease in hot flashes, with total number of hot flashes decreasing even more each week of the study.[1]

Improves mood and memory

Researchers noted in a study on Alzheimer's disease that sage has been used in herbal medicine for centuries to improve mood and cognitive performance. In studying the herb on patients in Iran, they found that sage produced significantly better outcomes in disease management than a placebo, and may also be responsible for reducing agitation in the patients.[2]

1. Bommer, S., et al. "First time proof of sage's tolerability and efficacy in menopausal women with hot flushes," *Adv Thera* 2011 Jun; 28(6):490-500. http://www.ncbi.nlm.nih.gov/pubmed/21630133

2. Akhondzadeh, S., et al. "Salvia officinalis extract in the treatment of patients with mild to moderate Alzheimer's disease: a double blind, randomized and placebo-controlled trial," *J Clin Pharm Ther* 2003 Feb; 28(1):53-9. http://www.ncbi.nlm.nih.gov/pubmed/12605619

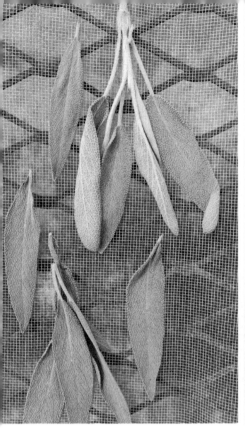

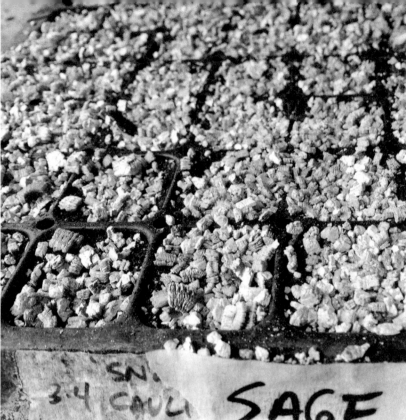

Left: Sage leaves drying on a screen.

Right: Using vermiculite after planting can keep the seeds warm and cozy for germination.

VARIETIES Sage boasts dependable, hearty leaves that dry like a charm. In early summer, small edible flowers appear that can also be added to dishes or teas. Usually, when buying sage at a store, you're likely to get common sage, a familiar variety that has a uniform look, but there are others worth trying as well. Check out these, all with good medicinal properties:

- **White Sage:** A Native American variety that's often used to make smudge sticks that are burned in ceremonies. Makes a mild-tasting tea, and grows well in warmer climates.
- **Berggarten:** Features oval leaves rather than the oblong leaves seen with other sage varieties. Purple edible flowers in early summer.
- **Extrakta:** Considered a high-yielding variety that can thrive in cooler zones. High essential oil content.
- **Icterina:** A newer variety with variegated leaves of green and yellow that makes a striking ornamental edible, especially in early season when edible purple flowers are present.

PLANT It isn't too difficult to get sage started indoors, but it's prone to death by overwatering. There have been many times where I see those tough leaves and think the plant looks dry, and then I end up killing it because it's already well-watered. Also, many experts advise waiting a long time before harvesting while the plant gets established—up to a year in some cases. For me, the space in my kitchen growing area is too limited to nurse a plant that takes months before I can use it, but I do like to have a small pot going because the herb dries so well after harvest.

The best way to grow sage is from cuttings from an established plant, so if you happen to have any neighbors or friends with a robust sage plant, see if you can sweet talk them into helping you out. The best time to get cuttings is from July to September, after the flowers have already come and gone.

Use a sharp knife to cut a young shoot well below the leaf crown. Strip off lower leaves, leaving at least three pairs of leaves. Put the shoot into a pot with new soil that's been worked with compost and water thoroughly but carefully so you don't displace the shoot. As the sage is establishing, make sure soil stays moist but not soaked. When the cutting seems to be growing and maturing you can transplant outside or put into a larger pot for an indoor kitchen garden.

Alternately, put the cutting into a glass of water, making sure the leaves are above the water line. After a few weeks, you'll begin to see roots, and the shoot can then be planted directly into a garden or a container. This is a fun activity for kids, since it allows them to see some progress on root growth.

If you're lacking access to established sage and want to start from seed, consider starting the seeds in a shallow container (about 2 inches or so) first, which will keep the roots warmer, aiding in germination. As the plant grows larger, transfer to a larger container (at least 6 inches deep) so the roots can establish more firmly. Whether the herb will be indoors or in a garden, put a small amount of slow-release fertilizer into the soil at the start of the season.

GROW Once it's established in a garden, sage is easy to maintain, and benefits from frequent harvesting, which encourages more growth. Just be sure to water younger plants more regularly so they don't dry out, but in general, when plants are more mature, wait until the soil seems dry before watering so they don't get root rot.

Sage can be subject to some pest and disease issues like aphids, powdery mildew, and stem rot, but these can be prevented by avoiding overwatering. If a plant does develop issues, remove the affected plant if the others around it seem fine. Otherwise, there are some organic pest sprays that can help, which are found at any nursery or greenhouse.

HARVEST & STORE During sage's first year, the herb won't be as robust as it establishes, so harvest lightly to give it a chance to expand. You can cut it back in late summer, but leave some stalks so the plant can come back strong the following spring. When harvesting, make sure leaves are clean; sage tends to pick up dirt, so I usually rinse them thoroughly and pat dry with a clean cloth before drying or using.

Use fresh sage for cooking or make an infused olive oil—simply drop some leaves into a bottle of oil and seal securely; store in a cool, dry place for a week and then place in the refrigerator. The oil will keep longer if you use dried herbs, but I tend to prefer the flavor of fresh leaves in infused oil. Olive oil boasts its own medicinal powers, since bacteria can't thrive in it, making it a good base for a remedy.

For teas and infusions, place cleaned leaves on a mesh screen and allow to dry completely before grinding or crumbling, then store in an airtight glass jar.

NUTRITIONAL VALUE OF SAGE

per 100 g (3.5 oz)

Sage is rich in vitamin A, vitamin K, potassium, and calcium.

Energy	315 kcal
Carbohydrates	60.73 g
Dietary fiber	40.3 g
Fat	12.75 g
Protein	10.63 g
Water	7.96 g
Vitamin A	5900 µg
Thiamine	0.754 µg
Riboflavin	0.336 mg
Niacin	5.720 mg
Vitamin B$_6$	2.690 µg
Folate	274 µg
Choline	0 mg
Vitamin C	32.4 mg
Vitamin E	7.48 mg
Vitamin K	1714.5 µg
Calcium	1652 mg
Iron	28.12 mg
Magnesium	428 mg
Manganese	0 mg
Phosphorus	91 mg
Potassium	1070 mg
Sodium	11 mg
Zinc	4.70 mg

Source: USDA Nutrient Database

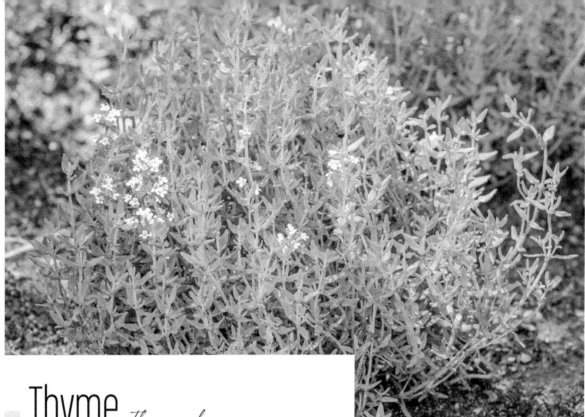

Thyme *Thymus vulgaris*

Although thyme's fragrance and flavor are associated with culinary efforts like pasta sauce and cooked meats, the plant's wee leaves have a rich history when it comes to symbolism. In the Middle Ages, the herb was thought to ward off nightmares if tucked under a pillow, and was often placed on coffins to help souls find their passage to the next life. That's likely why the ancient Egyptians used thyme for embalming as well. Apart from that maudlin usage, dried thyme—much like dried sage—has been utilized through the ages as a purifying agent, with smudge bundles burned in temples and homes. These days, it's recognized for a powerful active compound, thymol, which is often used in mouthwashes and as an antiseptic in hospitals.

Thyme is very potent as an essential oil, and in that form, it's been used to medicate bandages, treat infected toenails, and perform other anti-fungal medicinal tasks, although it also boasts anti-inflammatory and anti-bacterial properties.

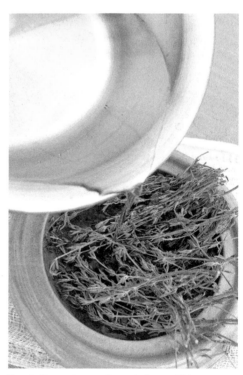

Pour boiling water over thyme to be used later for preparations.

The herb is also a standout for its ability to treat coughs and bronchitis as a tea, and also does well when combined with other medicinal plants like lemon balm.

Here are a few ideas for your Rx/medicinal preparations:

- For a nice addition to cough remedy teas, pack fresh thyme into the bottom of a jar and pour honey over the top; stir herbs into the honey and wait about a week for the infusion to "take." Strain the herbs out, or include them with the honey when adding to hot water or tea.

- Make a poultice by mashing fresh leaves into a paste; apply directly to rashes, minor sores, or other inflammation, with a clean cloth over the paste.

- Crush fresh leaves slightly and put into a small jar, and cover with vodka or vinegar that still contains "the mother" (such as Bragg's) as a preservative. Let the mixture sit at least overnight, and longer if possible; this mix works well as a mouthwash or antifungal wound wash.

PLANT·GROW·HARVEST·USE

As a perennial, thyme is a favorite in backyard pharmacy gardens because it's so hardy and keeps coming back strong. Unlike herbs in the mint family, thyme doesn't get to be a bully in the garden, but

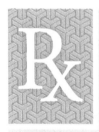

MEDICINE CABINET

Thyme is useful for a range of maladies, from bad breath to soothing muscle spasms. The herb (like so many others) has been noted as a hangover remedy, but it shines brightest for skin treatments, and Hippocrates noted its value for respiratory issues.

Better for acne than prescriptions

Researchers from Leeds Metropolitan University studied the effects of thyme, marigold, and myrrh on a certain type of acne that stems from infected skin pores, and found that thyme was not only the best of the three, but also boasted a greater antibacterial effect than benzoyl peroxide, the active ingredient in most anti-acne medications.[1]

As effective as ibuprofen for menstrual pain

In studying dysmenorrhea, in which women experience significant pain during menstrual cycles, researchers at Babol University of Medical Sciences in Iran found that thyme essential oil was equally effective at reducing pain and spasms as ibuprofen, but didn't cause the type of gastrointestinal complications sometimes seen with ibuprofen.[2]

1. Society for General Microbiology. "Thyme may be better for acne than prescription creams." ScienceDaily. 27 March 2012. www.sciencedaily.com/releases/2012/03/120327215951.htm
2. Salmalian, H., et al. "Comparative effect of thymus vulgaris and ibuprofen on primary dysmenorrhea: A triple-blind clinical study," *Caspian Journal of Internal Medicine* 2014; 5(2):82-88. http://www.ncbi.nlm.nih.gov/pmc/articles/PMC3992233/

instead stays fairly self-contained, bushy and tall instead of gangly and sprawling. Outdoors, thyme can tolerate drought, light freezes, and strong winds, so boasts a surprisingly long growing season after being planted in the spring. This is a nice choice for indoor growing as well, and can be included in a pot with other herbs like sage or basil.

VARIETIES The type of thyme found most often in medicinal preparation and cooking is German thyme, a hearty and dependable variety that's as robust as a Frankfurt beer hall. Because of its bushy shape and needle-shaped evergreen leaves, the herb variety often makes a nice ornamental, particularly along walkways or alongside flowers. For a wider range of options, though, there are other varieties that are equally useful. Although these all have distinct culinary properties, they're also powerful medicinals:

- **Orange Thyme** or **Lemon Thyme:** With the classic thyme shape, these varieties are also ideal for indoor growing and outdoor herb spaces, and have a sweeter flavor than the rugged German variety. A citrus flavor note makes the varieties a good choice for fish and vegetable dishes, or a distinctive honey-and-thyme mix.
- **French Thyme:** *Tres bien* for culinary dishes, although the flavor is more subtle than the German option. The variety is low growing, so it's perfect for smaller spaces, and the leaves are more round and soft than spiky and needlelike.
- **Creeping Thyme:** If you're looking for an ornamental plant, this variety works well in warmer climates, and features rounded leaves that "creep" out as a groundcover. Bonus: it can withstand light foot traffic, and gives off a thyme-infused scent when you walk on it.

Strip leaves off after you've dried the thyme.

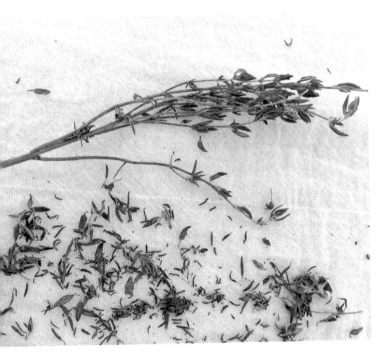

PLANT Thyme can be direct-seeded into a garden, if you have just the right conditions for it, but it thrives best if it's transplanted from a start that's been nurtured indoors for at least a month. Either buy a small start from a greenhouse, or grow one yourself in a warm and cozy indoor space in early spring for planting after the last frost.

If growing outside, pick a spot with full sunshine and soil that drains well. Compacted soil will result in slow growth, or even no growth at all, so if your chosen thyme spot seems dense, loosen up the area with a pitchfork or other cultivating tool.

For inside growing, consider starting the seeds in a small container (about 2 inches or so) first, which will keep the roots warmer, aiding in germination. As the plant grows larger, transfer to a larger container (at least 6 inches) so the roots can

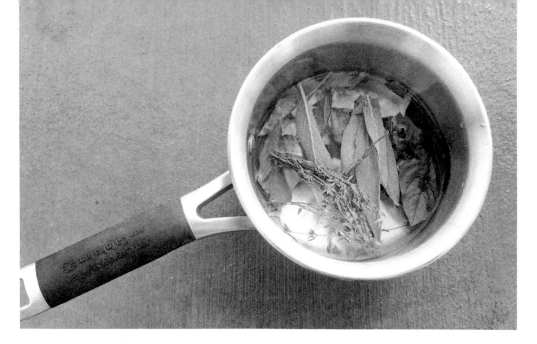

Thyme combines well with other herbs and medicinals.

NUTRITIONAL VALUE OF THYME

per 100 g (3.5 oz)

Thyme is rich in folate, choline, vitamin E, vitamin K, calcium, iron, magnesium, zinc, and potassium.

Energy	1156 kJ (276 kcal)
Carbohydrates	63.94 g
Dietary fiber	37 g
Fat	7.79 g
Protein	9.11 g
Water	92.06 g
Vitamin A	190 µg
Thiamine	0.0513 µg
Riboflavin	0.399 mg
Niacin	4.940 mg
Vitamin B_6	0.550 µg
Folate	274 µg
Choline	43.6 mg
Vitamin C	50.0 mg
Vitamin E	7.48 mg
Vitamin K	1714.5 µg
Calcium	1890 mg
Iron	123.6 mg
Magnesium	220 mg
Manganese	7.867 mg
Phosphorus	201 mg
Potassium	814 mg
Sodium	55 mg
Zinc	6.18 mg

Source: USDA Nutrient Database

establish more firmly. Whether the herb will be indoors or in a garden, apply a small amount of slow-release fertilizer into the soil at the start of the season.

Sometimes, thyme and other herbs can struggle if the pH of the soil is off, so in that case, test your soil to make sure it's alkaline enough for the thyme; it should be at about 7.0. If it's lower, boost it with a little lime sprinkled around the base of the plant.

GROW Like many herbs, thyme does well with frequent harvesting, which encourages more growth, especially during the summer. When done with the harvest season (which will depend on your particular growing zone) just let it flower so that it can keep going strong for the next year, but be sure to trim the plant back after flowering so that it doesn't get woody with overly thick stems. Over the winter, either pot it up to bring the plant inside to continue its growth, or protect it from deep freezes by covering it in the garden.

In terms of maintenance, thyme is an easygoing addition to the backyard pharmacy mix, and doesn't require much care beyond occasional watering. If the plant seems to be struggling, either move it to a sunnier spot, or try cultivating around the base so that the soil loosens for better drainage.

HARVEST & STORE Because thyme is a hearty, prickly kind of herb and not a delicate princess of a plant, you can harvest anytime of day (as opposed to late morning-only harvest for flowering and leafy herbs). Harvest frequently, since this encourages more growth.

In the summer, I prefer to use fresh thyme for remedies and medicinal preparations, since the flavor and aroma are stronger. When combined with lavender, for example, thyme becomes a pick-me-up aromatherapy choice.

But for use in the winter, thyme dries exceedingly well when stems are clipped, tied together in a bundle, and hung up to dry. Bundles can be stored in this form or stripped of their leaves and placed in small jars for use in cooking, teas, and even small sachets that can freshen the scent of drawers and closets.

For cooking, simply chop up the dried or fresh leaves and add to dishes, or bundle the leaves together with sage and bay leaves to make a bouquet garni, used to make an amazing soup stock.

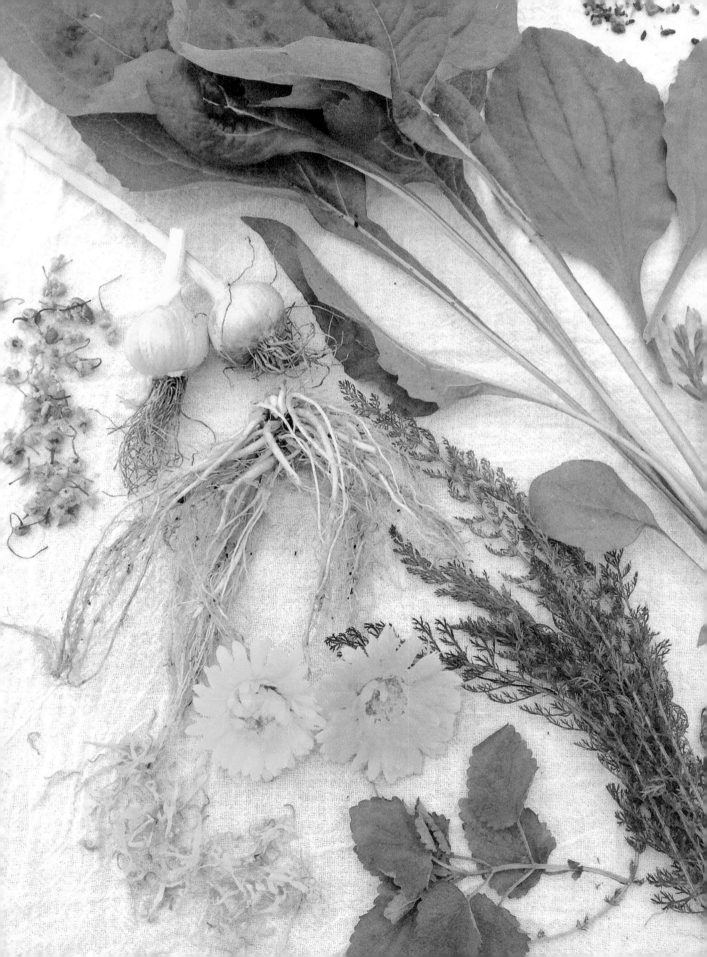

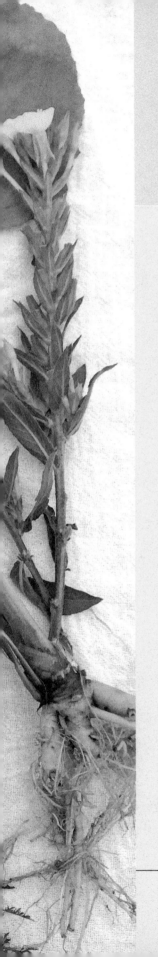

FOUR

Herbal Garden Remedies

With the exception of early experiences—creating "potions" in the culvert of my elementary school— I've felt somewhat intimidated by medicinal herbs, even though I've long been a fan of complementary medicine and alternative therapies. I could expound on the advantages of acupuncture and reiki, but when it came to using echinacea, I was clueless.

Going to herbal healers was beneficial, but I never dreamed that I could replicate those complicated mixtures. When I quit smoking and developed chronic respiratory issues during the detox period, a brilliant herbalist created a concoction with coltsfoot, mullein, hyssop, licorice, and something called mouse ear that I really hoped wasn't what it sounded like. Although it worked well, I still didn't consider making my own remedies; it felt similar to trying to create my own prescriptions. Who can whip up penicillin in her kitchen?

Then I became a farmer, and started growing all kinds of vegetables I'd never eaten before. A small culinary herb patch expanded, including herbs that attract pollinators, such as calendula and chamomile. Not wanting to waste these, I prepared them for medicinal use, feeling at first that I was, indeed, trying to whip up homemade antibiotics.

Happily, it was easy. I use valerian to sleep better, arnica for insect bites, and yes, echinacea to knock out cold symptoms. Although I haven't quite gone from clueless to confident, I am adventurous, and that's a very nice place to be. The following are some of my favorite herbs, selected for stress-free growth and effective medicinal treatments. Rock on, fellow herbalists.

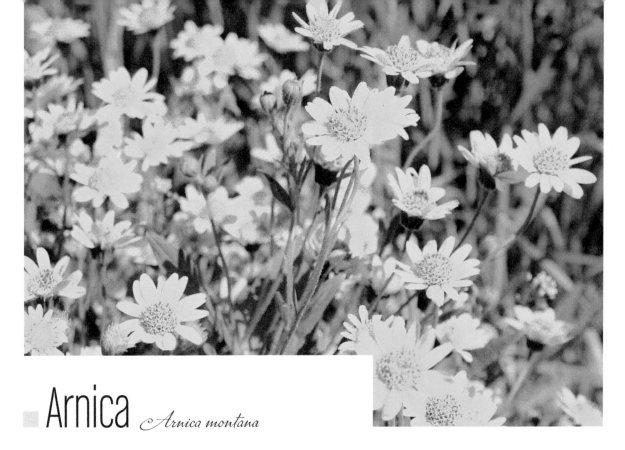

Arnica *Arnica montana*

From June to October, I use arnica almost every day, because it seems like I have some nightly complaint—sore shoulders from weeding all day, mosquito bites that stay itchy for hours, dry lips and hands—that could use some arnica love. The herb has been used for just such medicinal purposes since the 1500s, and there are plenty of preparations found in any natural remedies section of a co-op or grocery. Homeopathic practitioners use arnica for specific anti-inflammatory purposes, but in general, the herb is used topically since some serious side effects have been noted when used internally. The herb's name is likely taken from the Greek word *arna* (meaning "lamb") in reference to the plant's slightly hairy, soft leaves, even though all herbal preparations use only the flowers and not those lamb-like leaves.

Although herbs taken internally in the form of teas or essential oils shouldn't be used on a constant basis, those used externally like arnica

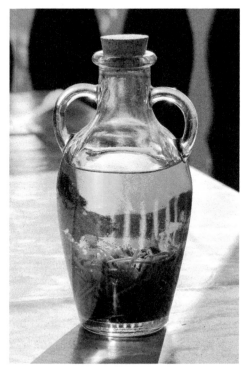

A tincture of arnica flowers and alcohol, placed in a sunny spot.

don't carry that caution. So, if you have nagging muscle pain or chronic issues like arthritis, try using arnica as a way to soothe those problems.

Here are a few ideas for your Rx/medicinal preparations:

- Create a tincture by pouring vodka (or other alcohol at least 70 proof) over freshly picked flowers. Seal tightly and let stand for at least a week in a sunny spot or warm area. Filter, put in a well-sealed container, and store out of direct sunlight.
- Combine the tincture with distilled witch hazel, which will increase the medicinal properties of your mix.
- Blend the tincture with a non-scented lotion or coconut oil for a topical lotion that will be moisturizing as well as soothing. If you can find some at your co-op, try using emu oil, since it has transdermal properties, which means it allows the herbal remedy to absorb more fully into the skin.

PLANT·GROW·HARVEST·USE

In addition to being a well-loved medicinal plant for bruises, aches, and pains, arnica is a happy little plant, bursting with bright yellow flowers thanks to its relation to the sunflower family. The plant grows to about 1 or 2 feet, with bright green leaves and a slightly hairy stem. They're seriously

CHECKLIST

Sun: Six to eight hours per day

Shade: Prefers full sun, but tolerates partial shade

Soil: Well-drained, loosened soil

Fertilizer: Once per season, sprinkle around roots

Pests: Tend to be minimal

Water: Regularly, depending on soil dryness

Grow Indoors? Yes

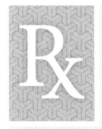

MEDICINE CABINET

Best known for easing pain and swelling from bruises, arnica is also used for aches, sprains, and even arthritis. Although it can be ingested, the herb is particularly ideal for any skin issues, from chapped lips to insect bites.

Helps bruises fade faster

In a small study on patients who had bruises created on their arms, researchers looked at four topical agents—vitamin K, retinol, arnica, and white petroleum—to study the speed of improvement. The rate of "bruise resolution" was significantly greater with arnica than with the petroleum, and also better than with the vitamin K and retinol.[1]

As effective as ibuprofen for osteoarthritis of the hands

In studying patients with osteoarthritis of the interphalangeal joints, researchers found that arnica gel was as effective as ibuprofen gel for treatment of pain, morning stiffness, and hand function. The study concluded that arnica could be used as an alternative to the commonly prescribed ibuprofen remedy.[2]

1. Leu, S., "Accelerated resolution of laser-induced bruising with topical 20% arnica: a rater-blinded randomized control trial," British Journal of Dermatology. 2010; 163: 557-563. http://www.ncbi.nlm.nih.gov/pubmed/20412090

2. Ross SM. "Osteoarthritis: a proprietary Arnica gel is found to be as effective as ibuprofen gel in osteoarthritis of the hands," Holistic Nursing Practice. 2008; 22: 237-239. http://www.ncbi.nlm.nih.gov/pubmed/18607237

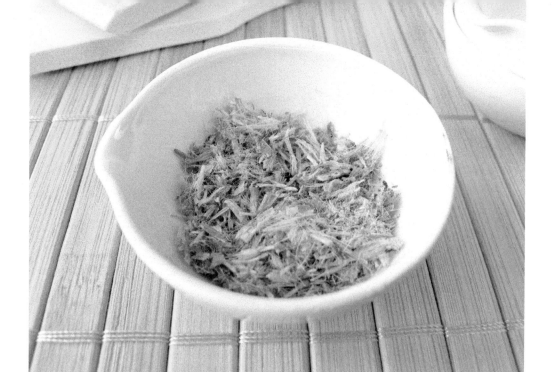

Dried arnica ready for using in a tincture.

adorable, and look a bit like wildflowers, so they're a nice choice for giving landscaping a softer, abundant look. Although they can be grown indoors, the flowers do well outdoors and are hardy in a range of climates—there are even some who grow them at over 8,000 feet in the Rocky Mountains. Because of its popularity, there are several areas of the world where harvesting wild arnica is illegal, including Italy, France, and the Ukraine, so cultivating it instead of foraging is the responsible choice.

VARIETIES Although arnica does have several varieties within the family, and boasts a few other names like mountain tobacco and leopard's bane, it's likely that when ordering seeds, you'll find only "mountain arnica" as a choice. Don't feel slighted by the lack of selection—this variety tends to be the hardiest and more predictable when it comes to growing. However, it's possible you may encounter other varieties like meadow arnica, and if you do, snap them up.

PLANT Arnica seeds first need to chill in order to germinate. This sounds counterintuitive to gardeners in warmer climates—doesn't refrigeration slow growth?—but the herb does best in higher elevations and temperate conditions, which tend to be cold right before natural germination periods. To mimic this, plant the seeds in small pots filled with peat moss and refrigerate or place in a cold frame for two to three months before transplanting out to their garden spot; aim for about 55 degrees Fahrenheit.

Sure, it's a super picky way to garden, and it can be annoying if you decide in May that you want arnica in your herb mix and realize that you missed your refrigeration window. But I've tried to skip this step before and ended up with greenhouse trays of soil that look like I forgot to plant in them.

If the refrigeration option is too fussy, then sow seeds outdoors in the late summer so they can come up the following year. But mark where you planted them, because sometimes they can take up to two years to grow with that particular method.

Once you do get the plants going and transplant outside, the good news is that arnica tolerates a range of soil conditions and climate types. In general, though, the herb prefers well-draining soil so be sure to cultivate well before planting. They also thrive in alkaline soil, with a pH range between 6.0 and 8.0, which can be adjusted by sprinkling agricultural limestone prior to planting.

GROW Choose a garden spot that gets some shade if you're in a warmer climate—the herb does well with full sun and blooms best that way, but it doesn't do well in dry, drought-type settings, so partial shade will provide some relief. The soil should be evenly watered to keep a nice degree of moisture, but not overly wet, which could lead to root issues.

If you've struggled with establishing arnica in a garden in the past, consider planting in a pot so you can control the herb's conditions better. That way, if it seems to be struggling in full sunlight, shift to partial shade. Alternately, if its shady location means that few blooms are popping, give it some much-needed sunshine.

When you have a nice patch going, it's easy to expand your arnica empire by dividing them up; just dig up part of the plant with roots, plant in a separate location and water well. If the plants have withered for the season, that's fine—you just need the rhizome anyway, which is the part of the rootstock that includes the little shoots from its sides.

HARVEST & STORE When I was a kid, we played a maudlin game with dandelions, in which we flicked off the blooms and called it "popping off the heads." When harvesting herbs like arnica, I think about this little second-grade practice almost every time—shout out to Sunnyside Elementary School!—since only the flowers are harvested. The roots can be used in some preparations, but for the most part, you're popping those heads.

In the summer, I prefer to use fresh arnica for remedies and medicinal preparations, since it's easy to make a tincture in just a week. Also, I tend to combine with calendula flowers to create a powerful herbal combo that can steep in alcohol on my windowsill. Once it's steeped as a tincture, either seal well and store in a cool place, or strain out the plant material and combine with lotion, oil, beeswax, or some other herbal preparation material.

Although a tincture will last practically forever, it's useful to dry some of the blooms for making preparations later. For that, use a clean metal or plastic screen, such as a fine-mesh cooling rack for baking, and evenly space the flowers for drying, away from insects and strong breezes. Once dried, pack into a jar and seal tightly, out of direct sunlight.

Fresh arnica blossoms are easy to dry, then make into a preparation.

NUTRITIONAL VALUE OF ARNICA

The nutritional value of arnica has not been established.

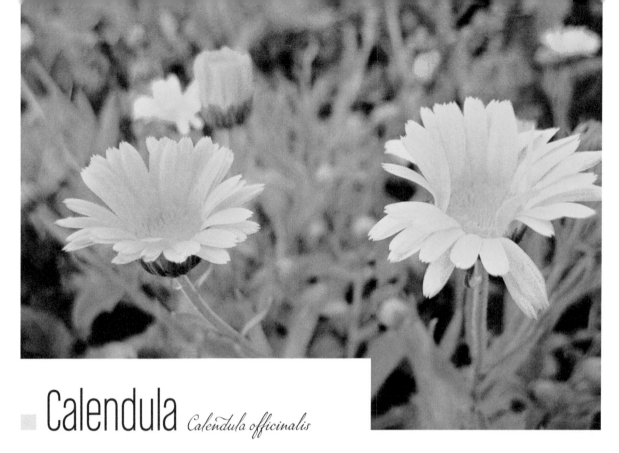

Calendula *Calendula officinalis*

Also known as pot marigold or garden marigold, calendula originates from southern Europe and has been one of the most used herbs throughout history—and not just for its medicinal properties. Considered sacred flowers in India, the calendula blossoms have often been used to decorate Hindu statues, and the flowers were also included in many Greek and Roman ceremonies. In the Middle Ages, it was rumored that if a girl walked barefoot on calendula petals, she would suddenly be able to understand the songs of birds. (Note: I've tried it. Doesn't work.) The cheerful, bright yellow and orange flowers have also been employed to color cheese and dye fabrics, similar to saffron (but without the hefty expense). Since the flowers are edible, they can also add some pop to salads or other dishes.

Although calendula can be used to treat stomach problems and ulcers, and has been employed to relieve menstrual cramps, most often the plant is used for topical applications,

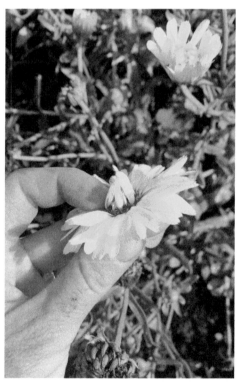

Harvest calendula by plucking the blossoms.

since it's so stellar at helping with skin and wound issues. According to the University of Maryland Medical Center, calendula has been shown to help wounds heal faster, possibly by increasing blood flow and oxygen to the affected area, so new tissue grows faster.

Here are a few ideas for your Rx/medicinal preparations:

- Place slightly wilted flowers (the quantity is not critical) in a jar with olive oil and put in a warm, sunny location, being sure to shake once a day to speed the infusion process; after a month, strain the oil and use for chapped skin, bruises, sore muscles, or diaper rash.
- Combine the infused olive oil with melted beeswax over a double boiler; once the wax is melted, you can stir in essential oils for scent if you like, but either way, pour into small tins or heat-resistant glass. Use the resulting salve for minor scrapes, insect bites, stretch marks, rashes, or chapped lips.
- Create a compress by pouring a cup of boiling water over a bowl of calendula flowers, covering, and letting the mix cool; strain out the flowers and soak a clean cloth in the water, then apply the compress to minor burns, insect bites, cuts, or bee stings until relief is felt.

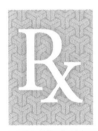

MEDICINE CABINET

Calendula is a powerhouse when it comes to skin treatments, and its effects are immediate rather than cumulative. Widely considered to be safe with some minor allergic reactions noted, the herb shows promise for a range of skin and wound issues, even in a clinical setting.

Prevents dermatitis during cancer treatment

A study published in the *Journal of Clinical Oncology,* and performed by radiation oncologists in France, found that patients receiving calendula had a significantly lower occurrence of acute dermatitis during radiation treatment, and many also reported reduced radiation-induced pain.[1]

Numerous healing properties

Researchers in India noted that calendula had been widely used in that country as a homeopathic medicine, so they broke the plant into its active chemical constituents to determine why it's so effective. They found a wide range of benefits, including anti-inflammatory, antibacterial, antifungal, and antiviral properties, and promising results for future research, calling the herb "future medicine for human kind."[2]

1. Pommier P, Gomez F, Sunyach MP, et al. "Phase III randomized trial of Calendula officinalis compared with trolamine for the prevention of acute dermatitis during irradiation for breast cancer," *Journal of Clinical Oncology* 2004;22:1447–53. http://jco.ascopubs.org/content/22/8/1447.full.pdf

2. Ukiya, M., et al. "Anti-inflammatory, anti-tumor-promoting, and cytotoxic activities of constituents of pot marigold (Calendula officinalis) flowers," *International Journal of Research in Pharmaceutical and Biomedical Sciences* 2006; 69:1692-96. http://www.ijrpbsonline.com/files/61-3294.pdf

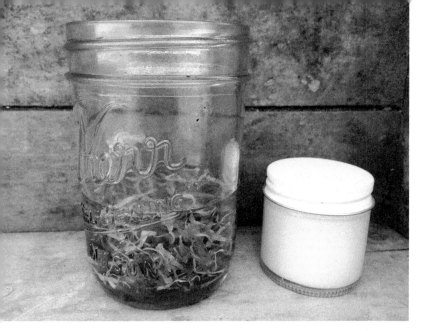

Calendula-infused oil to be turned into a balm.

PLANT·GROW·HARVEST·USE

Although some medicinal herbs and flowers can be fussy to grow (I'm looking at you, blue vervain), calendula is fairly easy, and can be either directly seeded right into a garden, or started indoors as transplants. Once they're established in a garden they'll self-seed so you don't have to keep replacing them every year, but they also won't become a nuisance by seeding heavily throughout their space. In other words, they're one of the "plays well with others" type of plants.

VARIETIES As a genus, calendula has about fifteen to twenty different species, and one particularly prevalent species is *Calendula arvensis,* also known as field marigold. Also seen across the world but originating in Europe, the arvensis grows wild in many areas. Other types, such as the sea marigold (*Calendula maritima*), are considered very rare and are actually endangered.

Although every species boasts lovely flowers, the type used most often for medicinal preparations, and the kind you'll want to grow in your garden, is *Calendula officinalis,* which has been more widely studied for its medicinal compounds. Within this type are several varieties, so you can choose blooms based on a wide color selection:

- **Alpha:** Happy, bright orange blooms will brighten up the garden, but the main benefit of this variety is the high resin content, which makes it more effective as a medicinal plant.
- **Indian Prince:** A two-tone variety that stands a little taller than many other options. The deep orange petals have a touch of crimson, and they're quite easy to start from seed.
- **Resina Calendula:** Although this variety has smaller flowers compared to some other types, it boasts the highest concentration of resins, giving it the most medicinal potency of any known calendula variety.

PLANT Because I live in the Midwest, where winters are approximately eighteen months long, I tend to prefer starting plants indoors in early spring, and nurturing them along until it's time to transplant them into the garden. Calendula does very well with this method, so if you have any kind of space where you can establish seed starts, you may want to consider giving the calendula this kind of head start. Otherwise, the plants will grow well if directly seeded into an outdoor garden space, and their ability to tolerate a mix of sun and shade make them a nice option for those tricky in-between landscaping spaces.

If growing inside, consider starting the seeds in a small container (about 2 inches deep or so) first, which will keep the roots warmer and cozier, aiding in germination. As the plant grows larger, transfer to a larger container (at least 6 inches deep) so the roots can establish more firmly. By the time it's about to outgrow that container, you can transplant outside.

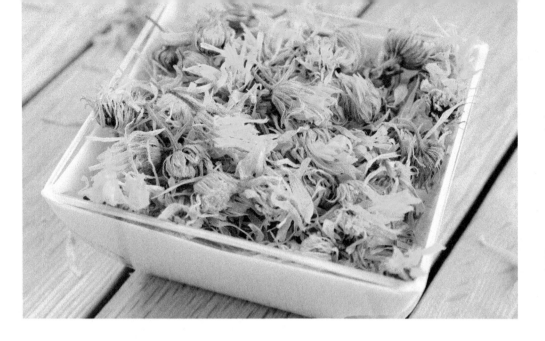

Dried calendula flowers being stored for later usage.

Whether you're direct seeding or transplanting, loosen the soil first to minimize compaction issues, and plant either in early spring or early fall, since the plants don't do as well in hot temperatures. If you're living in a particularly steamy area, consider a variety like Pacific Beauty Mixed Colors, which offers more heat tolerance.

GROW Because of its minimal maintenance needs and adaptability to different soil types, it's easy to see why calendula became so established across the world as a medicinal and decorative option. The roots can adjust to whatever space they're given, so you can grow calendula in a container, raised bed, or open garden space. The plants don't require fertilizer or abundant care, and they do well with a kind of benign neglect, as long as they're not in very hot conditions or left without water for long periods.

The only maintenance required is to deadhead the plant regularly, which means plucking the dead or faded flowers off the plant, a technique that helps it to thrive and stay blooming for longer. In the fall, keep some blooms going if you want the plant to self-seed for the next year.

HARVEST & STORE Much like many other types of flowers to be used for medicinal or edible use, calendula is best harvested in the late morning, after the dew has dried but before any warmth causes flowers to wilt or close. Don't be afraid to harvest frequently; cutting the blooms will encourage more budding, so you can get several rounds of flowers off one plant.

The flowers can be used fresh or dried, and if you prefer the latter, then place the flower heads on a screen in a shady spot that's warm but not hot. I've found that this method works best for flowers since it offers some airflow and prevents moisture issues. When they're dry and papery, store in canning jars or vacuum-sealed containers.

Drying is useful if you'd like to create ointments or oils in later months, but I tend to prefer using fresh flowers since medicinal preparation is so simple and quick (see Rx Medicine Cabinet for ideas).

Also, fresh flowers are edible, so anything I don't use for ointments can be added to dishes—keep in mind, though, that the petals are bitter, which makes it a good option for the digestion system, but also means that a little goes a long way.

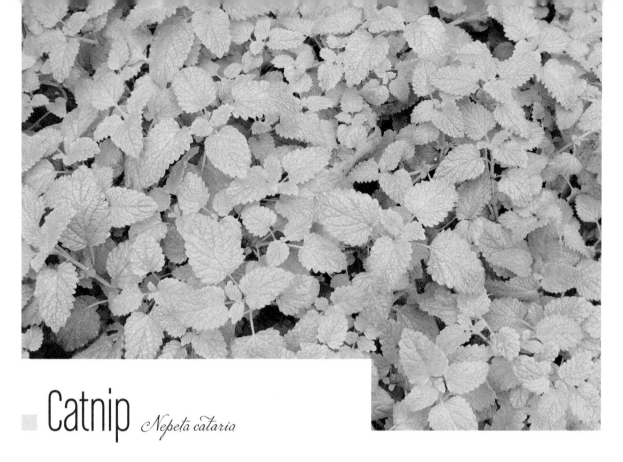

Catnip *Nepeta cataria*

Although most people think of catnip as a kind of kitty marijuana, the herb has been valued as a medicinal for humans since it was cultivated in Roman times—when the town where it was most cultivated, Nepeti, became part of its botanical name. The dried leaves were once smoked to relieve stress (much like non-kitty marijuana these days), and fresh leaves were utilized to reduce fevers, calm headaches, and soothe upset stomachs. In the United States, the herb isn't used very often except in cat toys for now, but in Europe, catnip is still used to tenderize and season meat. The herb's flowers, roots, stems, and leaves can all be used, making it a good all-around herb, and its mildly sedative effect is just as pleasant in people as it is for your mouser.

Although there's no clinical evidence to support use of catnip tea as a sedative, anecdotal reports abound about its use as a home remedy for reducing anxiety. Also, the tea has a very pleasant taste if prepared correctly.

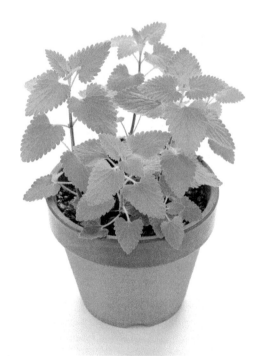

Putting catnip in a pot can keep it from spreading too much in a garden.

Here are a few ideas for your Rx/medicinal preparations:

- When making tea, use 1 teaspoon dried or 2 teaspoons fresh catnip (leaves or flowering tops). Boil water, but let it cool down slightly before pouring over the catnip, and steep for only about two to three minutes. Using boiling water and steeping for too long tend to make the tea bitter, but cooler water and a shorter steep produce a minty, complex taste.
- Make a poultice by mashing fresh leaves into a paste; apply to reduce fluid retention in the legs or to alleviate swelling or bruising until you feel relief.
- To help ease digestive troubles, fresh catnip can be used in culinary applications, such as chopped fresh into salads, or mixed with olive oil to create a tenderizing marinade for beef.

PLANT·GROW·HARVEST·USE

An easy-to-grow perennial, catnip is part of the mint family, and is sometimes called catmint, although there are some differences between the two species. Like other members of that family, catnip can get invasive if left unchecked, and spreads quickly. Most varieties reach about 3 or 4 feet, and feature large serrated leaves that often resemble nettles, but without that plant's prickly stems.

Even if you choose to use other herbs for anti-anxiety effects, there's always the option to grow catnip for the feline members of your family. The herb can be especially useful if you're fond of

CHECKLIST

Sun: Eight to ten hours per day

Shade: Prefers full sun

Soil: Well-drained, loosened soil

Fertilizer: Usually not necessary, the plant can do well with minimal intervention and inputs

Pests: Whitefly and spider mites; keep plants pruned to increase airflow

Water: When plants seem dry; don't overwater

Grow Indoors? Yes

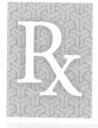

MEDICINE CABINET

Catnip hasn't been studied as extensively as other herbs, but hopefully that will change, given its potential for regulating digestion and soothing anxiety. But it has shown some promise in certain areas:

Repels mosquitoes better than DEET

The essential oil in catnip, nepetalactone, gives the plant a distinctive aroma, and it appears that mosquitoes hate the scent. In a presentation at the American Chemical Society, researchers noted that catnip is ten times more effective at repelling mosquitoes than DEET, the compound used in most commercial insect repellents.[1]

Rich medicinal history

Despite catnip's minor role in herbal remedies now, the herb actually boasted a wide range of uses in the past, according to a researcher who did a scientific literature review. He cited uses for hives, whooping cough, rheumatism, yellow fever, smallpox, and jaundice, as well as many other ailments.[2]

1. American Chemical Society. "Catnip Repels Mosquitoes More Effectively Than Deet." ScienceDaily. 28 August 2001. http://www.sciencedaily.com/releases/2001/08/010828075659.htm

2. Grognet, J. "Catnip: Its uses and effects, past and present," *The Canadian Veterinary Journal* June 1990; 31(6):455-456. http://www.ncbi.nlm.nih.gov/pmc/articles/PMC1480656/?page=2

growing plants indoors, since it can be strategically placed to distract cats from culinary herb pots and houseplants. Also, there's some evidence that catnip can repel fleas, so let your kitty loll around in the leaves all she wants. The more cats crush the plant (and they will, believe me), the more oil gets released, leading straight to kitty nirvana.

VARIETIES Catnip actually has a wide range of varieties, but when it comes to growing them, the options are fairly limited. Still, it's possible to do some research with seed companies and find lesser-known varieties. Here are some to consider:

- **Common Catnip:** When ordering seeds, if a variety isn't specified, it's most likely common catnip. Plants grow about 3 feet high, and leaves are a grayish green, with white flowers.
- **Camphor Catnip:** If you want to grow catnip for yourself instead of your cats, this variety is a good choice, since cats tend to avoid it. Also, its smaller size makes it more controllable in a garden.
- **Lemon Catnip:** Similar to common catnip in height and color, but the flowers have purple spots and the plant smells of lemon.
- **Greek Catnip:** A shorter variety at about 18 inches tall, this catnip has pale green leaves and pink flowers, also making a very pretty ornamental.

PLANT Catnip can be directly seeded into a garden space, but I've found that it's best either to purchase plants from a nursery or to start the plants indoors before transferring them to an outside space or a larger container. If you know someone who's already growing catnip, you can ask for a section of what they have and replant it in your own space. Just be sure to get roots as well as leaves and plant in well-loosened soil.

Whatever method you choose for your starts, pick a spot in full sun and water frequently so the catnip can fully establish. If you're trying to keep cats away from the space, consider using some fencing, bird netting, or other strategies that allow the plant to grow undisturbed.

Catnip can be a very versatile plant, and not just for kitties.

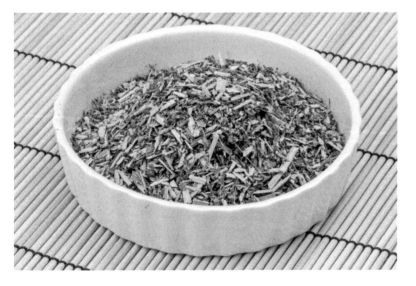

If starting from seed, sow in early spring or in the fall so it can overwinter and then germinate the next spring. This method tends to produce a denser crop of catnip, which can be nice if you're looking for abundance.

One of the best aspects about catnip is that it can thrive in poor soil, unlike some other herbs that require more nourishment. That makes catnip an ideal choice for areas where other plants might struggle, especially along walkway borders or in more alkaline soil.

GROW Like other types of mint, catnip can get invasive if you let it, so it's best to keep it trimmed back. You can also ensure a fuller

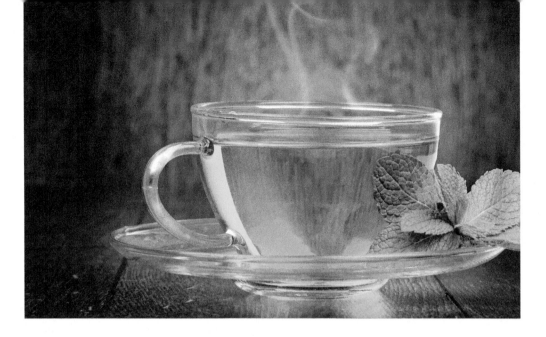

Catnip tea has a minty taste.

plant and less invasion by pinching off the flower buds when they first appear, but I tend to like a taller plant with plenty of pretty white flowers, so catnip is one of the wild things in my garden space.

Another way to keep control is to thin the plants when they're in an early stage, usually about 5 inches tall. Plants should be around 12 inches apart, so take out any that seem to be crowding closer than that.

If growing indoors, make sure the plants are getting enough light; if they don't, the herbs tend to get spindly. Also, be careful not to overwater or let the herb sit in water, since that can prompt root rot.

HARVEST & STORE Like many herbs, catnip is best harvested in late morning, after the dew has dried. This technique is especially helpful if you'll be using the catnip fresh, a nice idea if you're going to throw the leaves into a lunchtime salad. The leaves have a light, minty flavor, as long as you use younger, more tender leaves. Avoid the larger leaves as an edible, since they can sometimes taste grassy or woody.

Before adding a healthy amount to any dish or tea, try a leaf or two first to see if you have any adverse reactions. Most likely, this won't occur, but occasionally I find that I have minor sensitivities to fresh medicinal herbs. For example, I wouldn't load up a salad with fresh senna leaves, unless my digestive system needed a massive cleanse, shall we say.

As any cat owner knows, catnip dries beautifully, which is why it's so easy to tuck into little mouse-shaped toys. You can tie a bundle together and hang up to dry, or pick individual leaves and place on a mesh screen so they dry flat. I tend to prefer the latter method even though it's more time consuming, because I'm not a fan of crushing up bundled herbs that require an additional step of picking the stems and other non-leaf material out of the mix. (But if you're making cat treats instead of tea or tinctures, bundle drying and a rough crush is probably the way to go.)

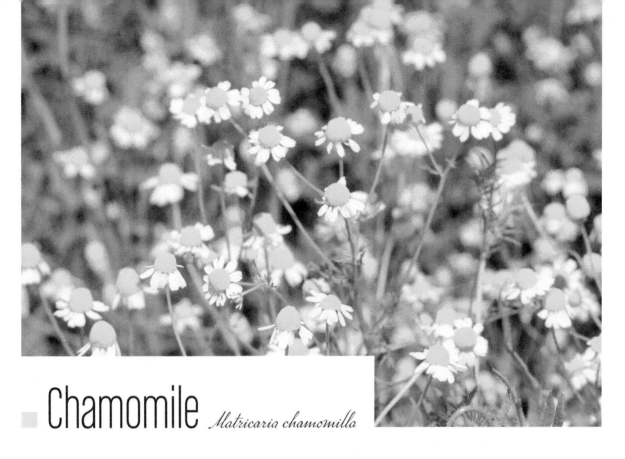

Chamomile *Matricaria chamomilla*

For a plant that's frequently found growing wild in poor soil, chamomile has an impressive pedigree. The ancient Egyptians dedicated the plant to their gods, since they considered the herb sacred, and numerous cultures have utilized the plant for its medicinal properties. The Greeks called the plant "Earth Apple" because they thought the scent smelled so fruitlike, and the herb is so hardy that it was once used as groundcover, similar to lawns.

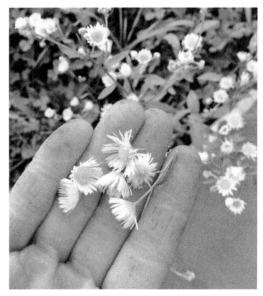

Chamomile flowers being harvested.

According to the National Institutes of Health (NIH), over one million cups of chamomile tea are consumed every day, and the NIH notes that the herb is one of the oldest, most widely used, and well-documented medicinal plants in the world. Try to remember that the next time you see it sprouting up next to your garbage can.

Although chamomile boasts a range of uses, it's most often used as a calmative, which means that it lowers anxiety and helps ease sleep issues. The herb is such a gentle sedative that many herbalists recommend it for children, and its anti-inflammatory properties can be helpful for digestive problems, sore throats, and tired eyes.

Here are a few ideas for your Rx/medicinal preparations:

- Create a decoction (see Chapter 2 for instructions) and pour into a warm bath; this is not only calming, but the herb's combination with the steam helps ease respiratory ailments.
- For gingivitis, pour a cup of boiling water over 3 teaspoons of the dried leaves and let infuse for five to ten minutes; after it cools, use as a mouthwash.
- Dry the flowers in a single layer on a clean mesh surface or cooling rack, then crumble and use as a tea for insomnia or general chill-out drink.

PLANT·GROW·HARVEST·USE

Cheery and resembling tiny daisies, chamomile often resembles a wildflower, with its feathery leaves and abundant blooms. Because it does well in a wide range of soil types, chamomile fills in well in garden spots that might not have the best soil for pickier plants. It's also considered an ideal companion plant to others because it helps to repel insects, which means that if you've had

CHECKLIST

Sun: Eight to ten hours per day

Shade: Prefers full sun but does well with partial shade

Soil: Well-drained, but tolerates a wide range of soil types

Fertilizer: Usually not necessary, the plant can do well with minimal intervention and input

Pests: Minimal

Water: Only during a long spell of hot weather, or when particularly dry

Grow Indoors? Yes

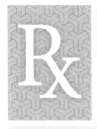

MEDICINE CABINET

Sometimes it seems that the list of what chamomile doesn't treat must be shorter than what it can address. It can't do your taxes, for example. Beyond that, it can probably address whatever is ailing you, from insomnia to wounds to indigestion.

Promise for a range of issues

Researchers from Case Western Reserve University note that chamomile flowers contain terpenoids and flavonoids that contribute to its medicinal properties, and preparations are commonly used for hay fever, anxiety, coronary heart disease, colic, hemorrhoids, and other issues. They noted that more clinical trials should be undertaken to discover all of its therapeutic benefits.[1]

Potential anti-cancer properties

Although chamomile has been used to treat a range of ailments, researchers noticed that its anti-cancer activity hadn't been evaluated. They exposed chamomile extracts to various human cancer cells, and found a significant decrease in cell viability with those cells, without negatively affecting normal cells. Researchers noted, "this study represents the first reported demonstration of the anti-cancer effects of chamomile."[2]

1. Srivastava, J., et al. "Chamomile: An herbal medicine of the past with a bright future," *Mol Med Report,* Nov 2010; 3(6):895-901. http://www.ncbi.nlm.nih.gov/pmc/articles/PMC2995283/#R53
2. Srivastava, J., Gupta, S. "Antiproliferative and apoptotic effects of chamomile extract in various human cancer cells," *Journal of Agricultural and Food Chemistry,* Nov 2007; 55(23):9470-8. http://www.ncbi.nlm.nih.gov/pubmed/17939735

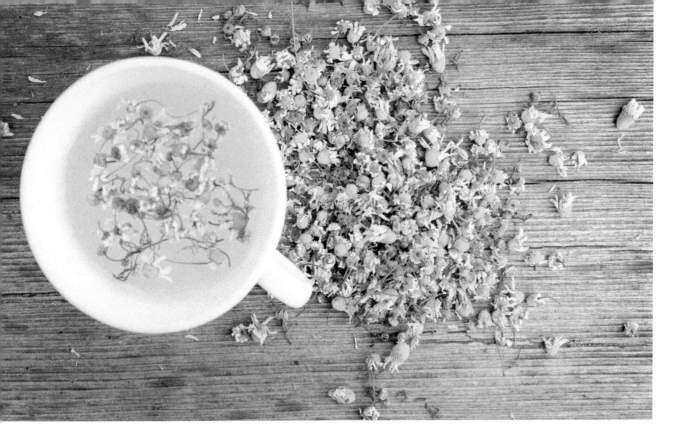

Dried chamomile makes a delicious and soothing tea.

aphid problems or cucumber beetles in the past, now's the time to let chamomile work its garden magic.

VARIETIES The type of chamomile found most often in medicinal preparation and from seed purveyors is German chamomile, a hardy annual that can grow up to 3 feet tall, and matures as a bushy shrub. The other common variety, Roman chamomile, is a perennial that only grows about a foot high. Although both have similar medicinal properties and can be used interchangeably, they have different growing needs. Most likely, when you see chamomile sprouting alongside roads and in sidewalk cracks, they're Roman. But if you want to cultivate some for your medicinal garden, I'd recommend German, since it tends to have more flowers, and those are what you use most for herbal preparations.

PLANT Although chamomile can be seeded directly into a garden, the herb tends to do best with a little head start. Plant indoors, about six weeks before you plan on transplanting it outside, and use smaller pots or trays at first to maintain warmth for the roots. When seeding, sprinkle a couple seeds in each pot, and don't cover with soil—the plant needs light to sprout, so blocking it will delay germination or even prevent it altogether. Once the seeds have started growing, thin them down to one plant per pot. Choose the hardiest; this is not a moment to root for the underdog.

Keep the seedlings in a sunny location until you plant them outside, or transfer the young plants into a larger container if you're planning on growing them inside. Chamomile does well as an indoor plant, especially if you have a sunny area by a window so it can get some airflow as well as light.

If direct seeding into a garden, plant seeds in the early spring, after the last frost, or even better, plant in the fall so that the seeds can overwinter and germinate the following spring.

Although German chamomile is an annual, it's likely that you won't have to replant every year since the herb is stellar at seeding itself as long as you allow some of the blossoms to go to seed. The plant is so effective at coming back year after year that it's a good idea to choose your chamomile spot wisely, since it's likely to become a long-term resident. Sometimes, it can be invasive and take over more than its allotted space, so if you want more control over the amount growing, try transplanting into outdoor pots.

GROW If growing indoors, you'll need to pay more attention to the plant than you would if it's outside in the garden, but not to a large degree. Just make sure the plant is in an appropriate-sized pot of at least 12 inches deep, containing some well-draining soil. If the herb seems slow growing or begins to yellow, transfer to a pot that has a better indoor soil mix, such as one that contains vermiculite or other drainage helper.

Outdoors, the plants won't require much care, which is one of the reasons I love growing it—I'm a big fan of benign neglect whenever possible (sorry, neighbors!). Occasionally the herb might start to struggle, and adding some fish-based fertilizer around the base can help especially at planting time. Otherwise, just water when it seems especially dry.

HARVEST & STORE Like other types of flowers, chamomile is best harvested in the late morning, after the early dew has dissipated but before the afternoon heat sets in. Because the flowers are quite small, it can take some time to harvest enough to turn into a medicinal remedy, especially since they shrink even more during the drying process. There's even a "chamomile rake" available online—resembling a deep dustpan with a comb on the bottom, the rake lets you harvest chamomile blossoms quickly. No matter what you're using, harvest in midsummer, when the flowers are most open.

Once you have the blossoms, lay them out in a single layer on a drying rack, such as a wood box frame with a fine plastic mesh. For some herbs, I use a kitchen cooling rack, meant for baked goods and cookies, but chamomile flowers are too small for this method, and I've found that something resembling a window screen is much better. Also, I prefer to air dry rather than put in a dehydrator, because the drying process is more even—otherwise, I get chamomile crumbles in the bottom of the dehydrator. However, there are some machines that have an "herb" setting that could be used for the effort.

When fully dry, pack into a glass jar, seal tightly, and keep in a dry, cool spot. Be sure to check on them in another week or so to determine if any mold or mildew is growing; if you find any evidence of that, you'll have to throw it out. Just be sure to dry the flowers for a longer time period next time.

NUTRITIONAL VALUE OF CHAMOMILE
The nutritional value of chamomile has not been established.

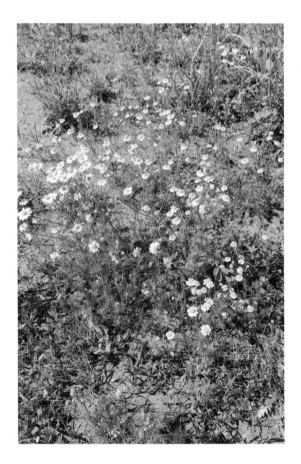

Once you plant or transfer chamomile, it can begin to grow wild.

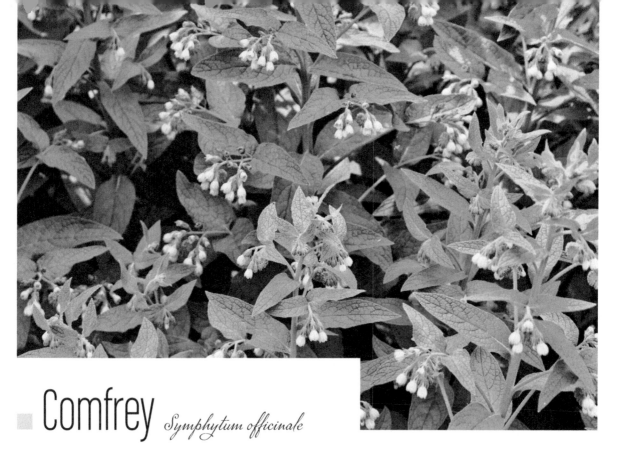

Comfrey *Symphytum officinale*

Native to Europe and some parts of Asia, comfrey is a perennial that features slightly hairy leaves and robust foliage, but it doesn't take over a garden space such as more impolite herbs like mint. At the end of its harvest season, comfrey sprouts pretty little flowers that begin with a blue hue but then fade to pink. The herb has long had a reputation for healing broken bones and acting as a general wound care go-to option, thanks to its high amount of allantoin, a substance that can boost healing by helping cell formation. Known to herbalists for over 2,000 years, comfrey was used in treating the wounds of Alexander the Great's army, and was in heavy use in the Middle Ages when it was cultivated by monks in their medicinal gardens.

Because comfrey has potential liver effects if taken internally, the University of Maryland Medical Center advises that you *do not* use comfrey on a child's skin, or use the herb for longer than ten days. Also, don't apply to broken

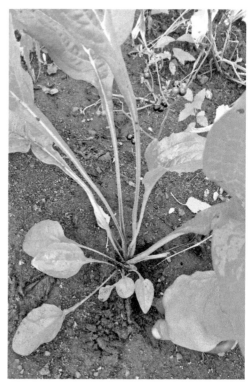

Comfrey roots can be dug up with just a small trowel.

skin. That's a great many caveats, but the herb is safe if used for topical applications of a few days, which is usually how long it takes bruises to heal with comfrey anyway.

Here are a few ideas for your Rx/medicinal preparations:

- Make a poultice by mashing fresh leaves with a mortar and pestle or a blender into a paste; apply directly to rashes, minor sores, or other inflammation, with a clean cloth over the paste. Be sure to put a warm towel (dipped into hot water and wrung out, or a dry cloth heated in an oven briefly) on top of the cloth, since heat can increase the effect of the allantoin.

- Crush fresh leaves and rub on blisters caused by poison ivy or poison oak (just be sure to avoid using on broken skin, which may have occurred from scratching).

PLANT·GROW·HARVEST·USE

As a perennial, comfrey is a nice choice for a medicinal herb garden since it comes back strong every year, and can be planted in spring, summer, or fall. It prefers well-worked soil with a pH of 6 to 7, but has also been known to do well in sandy or clay soil. Basically, it's adaptable to almost any situation,

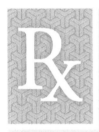

MEDICINE CABINET

Although comfrey was used in the past to address stomach issues, it was found that the herb has some substances, pyrrolizidine alkaloids, that can damage the liver, so several countries, including the US, have banned the sale of oral supplements. But the herb is still quite useful for topical applications, and stands out for its ability to help new skin cells grow, and to address sprains, bruises, and pulled muscles.

Helps with osteoarthritis

In a study examining the effects of comfrey on painful osteoarthritis of the knee, researchers found that those receiving topical comfrey showed significant improvement in pain management. They concluded that, "comfrey root extract ointment is well suited for the treatment of osteoarthritis of the knee. Pain is reduced, mobility of the knee improved and quality of life increased."[1]

Reduces back pain

Researchers found that the use of a cream that contains 35 percent comfrey root extract provided pain relief and more function to those who were suffering with acute upper or lower back pain.[2]

1. Grube, B., et al. "Efficacy of comfrey root (Symphyti offic. radix) extract ointment in the treatment of patients with painful osteoarthritis of the knee: results of a double-blind, randomised, bicenter, placebo-controlled trial," *Phytomedicine* 2007; 14(1): 2-10. http://www.ncbi.nlm.nih.gov/pubmed/17169543

2. Pabst, H., et al. "Combination of Comfrey Root Extract Plus Methyl Nicotinate in Patients with Conditions of Acute Upper or Low Back Pain: A Multicentre Randomised Controlled Trial," *Phytother Res.* 2012 Aug 8. http://www.ncbi.nlm.nih.gov/pubmed/22887778

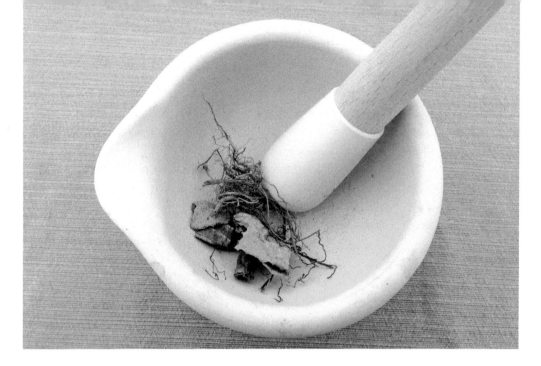

Roots and leaves blended together.

and can even thrive in partial shade. The herb grows in 120-degree African heat just as well as in the chilly Caucasus Mountains in Russia, and produces abundantly in both. You can even grow it indoors, as long as you commit to a large pot.

VARIETIES Comfrey comes in three main types: common, also known as Quaker or true, which grows 2 to 3 feet tall and can propagate through seeds; rough or prickly, native to Asia, considered invasive, and best propagated by roots; and hybrid or Russian, a cross between common and rough that grows up to 4 feet tall.

- **Bocking #4:** Considered a Russian variety, this comfrey is very hearty and has deep roots, making it ideal for drier climates.
- **Bocking #14:** Also Russian, this variety has the highest allantoin content, and is usually what's recommended for home gardens since the roots are more shallow, which means you can take them out if you switch up your garden plan.
- **Common:** The most cultivated variety, and hardier in cooler climates, down to Zone 3.
- **Red Comfrey:** Usually grown as an ornamental but still boasting medicinal properties, this variety has deep red flowers and is more compact than Russian or common varieties. It also has a nice shade tolerance.

PLANT The best system for planting comfrey can seem a little quirky, but it's much more fun than simply plunking a seed in the ground. So, let's start by talking about crowns and roots.

Comfrey is propagated with "crown cuttings," or root cuttings, which are basically sections of mature plants, and purveyors offer cuttings that are between one to twenty-five years old. Root cuttings look like dried cinnamon sticks, and are between 2 and 6 inches long. Dig a trench at least 2 inches deep, lay the cuttings flat, then cover with soil. Plant in the fall in order to get plants in the spring.

Crown cuttings are usually slightly more expensive, but can shorten the time between planting and germination. They're about 3 inches in length and look like gnarled, fairytale witch fingers (in my imagination, anyway) that have shoots or sprouts on one end. They're also planted flat, 3 to 6 inches deep, but with the sprouted end coming just above the soil surface or lightly covered with soil. Because the crown cuttings have sprouted buds already, they tend to be speedier in growing a full comfrey plant, and make a nice choice for planting in the spring.

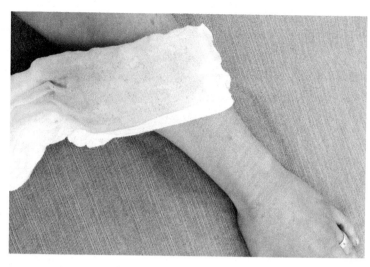

Comfrey made into a poultice after creating a paste.

Whichever you choose, comfrey cuttings do well with plenty of fertilization, so plan to work in azomite minerals, compost, rock phosphate, or other amendments into the soil before planting. Comfrey can tolerate higher levels of the nitrogen found in manure than any other plant in your garden, so if you're looking to use up some compost, comfrey will be happy to take it. Also helpful is to place plants in a grid pattern, about 3 feet apart, which allows easier harvesting.

For indoor growing, comfrey tends to do best in large pots or 5-gallon buckets, and crown cuttings are usually a good choice for getting results more quickly.

If you prefer to grow comfrey from seed then go for it, but keep in mind that it's not unusual to plant seeds and then not see any germination for at least two years.

GROW If you'd like to expand your comfrey empire, simply dig up some of the roots, and plant them in another part of the garden. Offer some to neighbors, put some on the breakroom table at work with some instructions, secretly plant some in an abandoned lot—let's make the world a comfrey-friendly place.

Comfrey requires minimal care, and gets a bit larger every year. Some plants can live for decades before they begin to decline.

HARVEST & STORE Comfrey grows about 12 to 18 inches tall and can be harvested almost down to the ground. Leave about 2 inches of growth, but otherwise just cut off the rest. Even with that aggressive cutting style, the plants should re-grow quickly so you can harvest again in two to four weeks. Just be sure to keep harvesting before the blooms appear, since the herb is at its most effective before that process begins.

In terms of storage, comfrey leaves tend to have higher moisture content than other types of herbs, which means they dry more slowly and are susceptible to mold if stored too soon. Avoid that risk by giving your comfrey a nice long drying period—for me, that often means hanging them in a dry, airy place and forgetting about them for at least a month. When the leaves are easily crumbled, that means it's ready for storage, so pack them into a well-sealed jar and store in a cool, dark place.

And seriously, don't eat it. If you have an herb book from the '70s, like several stars in my own collection, those authors recommend comfrey tea and make it sound heavenly—however, this was before significant research into the herb's effects on the liver. Topical only, please!

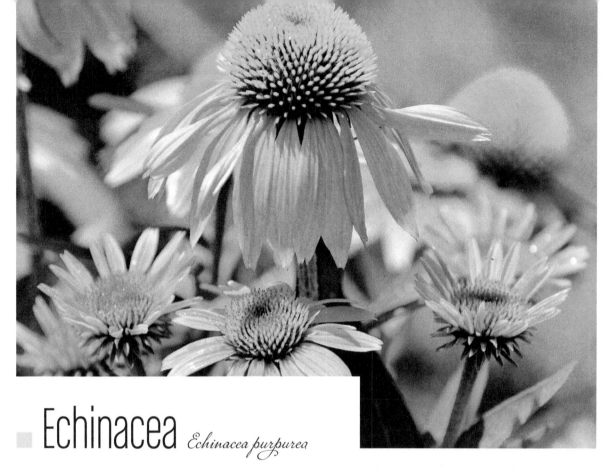

Echinacea *Echinacea purpurea*

A stunning plant, echinacea has been widely used for medicinal use by several tribes of North American Plains Indians. The herb's name comes from the Greek word *echino*, meaning *sea urchin*—so named because the coneflower that appears when it's mature resembles a spiny creature. (Fun note: there's a superorder of sea urchin called echinacea, distinctive because they possess gills, unlike most sea urchins. Currently, there's no evidence that using the herb echinacea will lead to gill formation, just in case you're wondering.) Regarding medicinal use, echinacea got trendy for cold relief, but study results are mixed when it comes to proof that it actually works for that. However, it does address some of the symptoms of a cold, such as sore throats, headaches, and coughs, and provides a strong boost to immune systems.

Echinacea has been widely used to address cold symptoms and upper respiratory

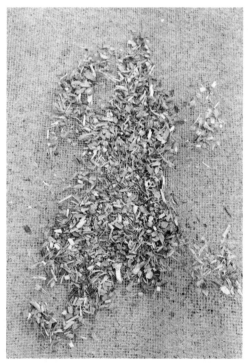

Echinacea shredded and drying.

issues, but the herb has numerous other uses as well, such as treating gum disease, chronic fatigue, migraines, and even rattlesnake bites.

Here are a few ideas for your Rx/medicinal preparations:

- For a general immunity boost, dry flowers and leaves, and then make into a tea; I tend to add other herbs for flavor, such as mint or holy basil.

- For a nice addition to cough remedy teas, take a moment in the summer to pack fresh echinacea flower petals into the bottom of a jar and pour honey over the top; stir herbs into the honey and wait about a week for the infusion to "take." Strain the herbs out, or include them with the honey when adding to hot water or tea. The mix will still be good all winter.

- Harvest roots in late fall, after the flowers have died, and dry on a screen in a well-ventilated location. When they're dry, make a decoction and drink as a warm beverage, sweetened with a bit of the flower honey, for shortening the duration of winter colds.

PLANT·GROW·HARVEST·USE

As a perennial, echinacea is a stunner in herb gardens because it's so distinctive and attractive. Although some species may sport different colors, the herb form is usually purple, and resembles

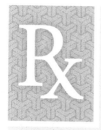

MEDICINE CABINET

Echinacea has become a nice cure-all kind of herb, helping the body fight infections, reducing pain and inflammation, and acting as an antioxidant. Herbalists might recommend echinacea for slow-healing wounds, sinus issues, antiviral remedies, and other treatments.

Enhanced immune function

Researchers looked at the effect of echinacea on T cells, which play a key role in the immune system. They found that supplementation with the herb led to enhanced immune function.[1]

Helps with cold symptoms

Whether echinacea knocks out a cold is still a matter of debate, but researchers found in one study that early intervention with a formulation of echinacea resulted in reduced symptom severity, especially with study subjects who had acquired an upper respiratory tract infection as a result of catching a cold.[2]

1. Kim, H.R., et. al. "Immune enhancing effects of Echinacea purpurea root extract by reducing regulatory T cell number and function," *Nat Prod Commun* 2014 Apr; 9(4):511-4.

2. Frank, L.G. "The efficacy of Echinacea compound herbal tea preparation on the severity and duration of upper respiratory and flu symptoms: a randomized, double blind, placebo-controlled study," *J. Comp. Alt. Med.* 2000; 6(4):327-334 http://www.ncbi.nlm.nih.gov/pubmed/14748902

a daisy. Echinacea also makes a good addition to garden spaces because it's easy to maintain, tolerates droughts fairly effectively, and can grow up to 4 feet tall, creating a nice border for landscaped spaces.

VARIETIES Echinacea is one of those plants that seem to inspire hybrid enthusiasts. The plant boasts nine distinct species, but more than fifty hybrids have been cultivated, creating different flower colors, more hearty varieties, and taller stems. There are some varieties, such as the yellow-flowered *Echinacea paradoxa,* that are considered rare, and a few others that are on the endangered list. For home planting, though, there are some good, dependable options that aren't likely to go missing anytime soon:

+ *Echinacea purpurea:* Considered the easiest to echinacea to grow, this variety does well growing from seed and has fibrous roots that are easy to harvest, as opposed to taproots that can be difficult to dig up.
+ *Echinacea pallida:* A taprooted variety with white pollen on the conehead; this tends to do well in cooler climates.
+ *Echinacea tennesseensis:* Sometimes, just planting an herb is an act of conservation, as is the case with this Tennessee coneflower. The plant is on the federal endangered species list, but seeds are available from a few online purveyors.

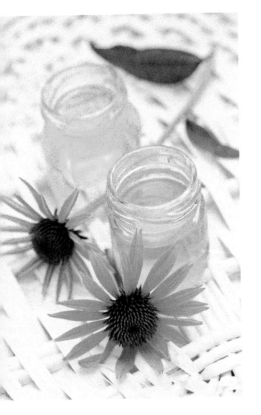

Echinacea flowers ready to be packed into jars of honey.

PLANT Echinacea can be direct-seeded into the soil with a variety like the *purpurea,* but germination is iffy at best. If you happen to know someone growing the plant, the best method to add it to your garden is through cuttings. This method is the most inexpensive, and for some herbs, is a perfect way to obtain a healthy plant that has a head start on growth. Simply dig up part of an existing echinacea patch, making sure to get as much of the root as possible—sometimes tricky, since the herb has a long taproot—and then plant in your space, making sure to water well so the transition won't be such a shock.

If you don't have a source for cuttings, plant seed instead, and opt for starting inside and transplanting to the garden later. Echinacea seeds tend to germinate quickly, usually in under a month, and you can nurture them along in your protected indoor space before putting them outside to establish. First, though, you usually have to cold stratify, which means mimicking the winter conditions necessary for a plant to emerge from winter's cooler temps.

To stratify, mix the seeds with a small amount of vermiculite or peat moss and sow into small containers. Then cover with plastic wrap to retain moisture, and place in a refrigerator kept under 60 degrees Fahrenheit. The seeds should germinate in about two weeks to a month, and then you can remove them and let them continue growing at room temperature.

Finally, you could also choose to buy starts from a greenhouse or nursery. Depending on where you live, this herb isn't always easy to find and may not be at large, conventional garden stores, but with its recent popularity, it's often available at specialty nurseries or smaller growers.

Wherever your source for transplants, choose a spot that gets full sun or is only partially in the shade, with soil that drains well and has a pH between 6 and 8. You can fertilize lightly with compost when transplanting, but in general, echinacea doesn't require fertilization once it's established.

GROW In terms of maintenance, echinacea is an easygoing addition to a garden, and doesn't require much care beyond occasional watering. The only time it seems to struggle is with too much rain or overwatering, since both can lead to root rot.

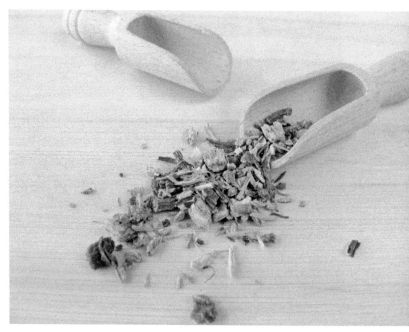

As the plants establish, be sure to keep them well-weeded, since weeds will provide too much competition for the plants. They won't get choked out by the weeds, but they could show slower growth, fewer blooms, and stunted stems.

If you live in a super chilly part of the world, as I do, you can tuck your echinacea in for the winter by covering the roots with a hay or straw mulch after the plants have died back and you've harvested any roots for your medicinal uses.

HARVEST & STORE Echinacea blooms are very pretty, especially when they're part of a prairie-like natural landscape, and they attract butterflies and birds. They also dry well when put on a clean screen or mesh surface. Just cut the flowers at the base, so you have only the flower head. You can also pick the petals and use those, leaving the seed-filled section behind for the birds.

The leaves can also be harvested by plucking, in order to dry those for tea and other preparations. As with other herbs, harvest is best in the late morning, when the morning dew has burned away but the afternoon heat hasn't set in yet.

If collecting roots, wait until October or November, when the plants have withered and there's been at least a first frost. This will cause the plant to divert its energy into the roots for winter storage, increasing their potency. Dry the roots in a cool, well-ventilated area until they can snap like twigs. After that, you can use in a decoction for an echinicea root tea.

Store roots, as well as dried leaves and flowers, in an airtight glass jar in a dark area, such as a cupboard, and consider it your winter cold knockout secret.

When dried, echinacea roots can be chopped up for long-term storage.

NUTRITIONAL VALUE OF ECHINACEA

The nutritional value of echinacea has not been established.

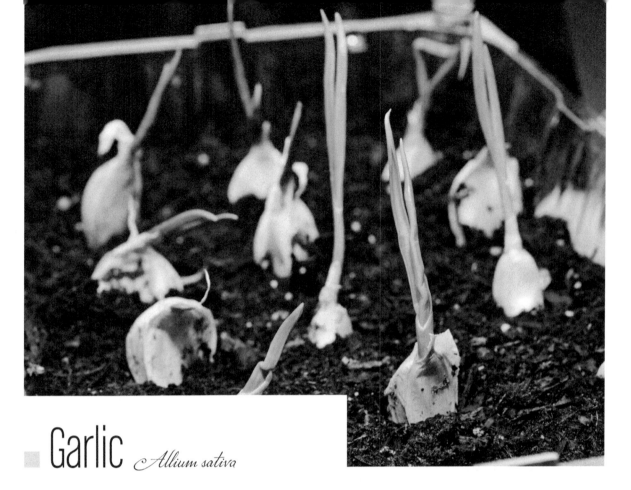

Garlic *Allium sativa*

When people ask how many fruits and vegetables we grow on the farm, I usually answer that we have about sixty, with several varieties within that. Occasionally, someone wonders which one is my favorite, and I don't even have to think about the answer: garlic. To me, and so many throughout history, garlic has been as close to a cure-all as you can get. A member of the onion family, garlic is native to Siberia, but is now grown in most of the world. Its use in folk medicine stretches back about 7,000 years, making it one of the oldest known medicinal foods or herbs. Some herbalists believe that even carrying a clove of garlic has some level of medicinal worth.

Garlic is favorite home remedy for many people, and shows promise as a remedy to reduce heart disease by lowering LDL

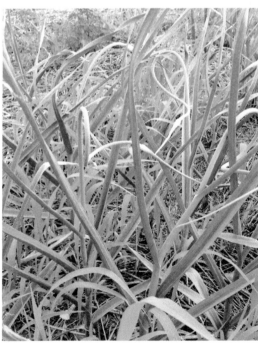

Garlic scapes, which appear about four weeks before harvest.

cholesterol. There's also some evidence that it can lower blood pressure, prevent blood clots, and address viruses and bacteria as well as parasites and fungi.

Here are a few ideas for your Rx/medicinal preparations:

- For colds and flu, cut up raw garlic and let sit for 15 minutes to release the allicilin, then swallow the small pieces with water, similar to taking pills. Repeat every few hours for an entire day; you'll start to sweat garlic, but this can significantly reduce the duration of a cold.

- For earaches, heat ¼ cup of olive oil and put about four chopped cloves into the pan, being careful not to boil the oil. Allow the mixture to cool down to a warm, but not hot, temperature and strain out the garlic. Put a few drops into the affected ear and let it sit about 10 to 15 minutes before tipping your head the other way to drain it back out.

- Treat warts by taking a slice of garlic and applying it directly to the wart, then rubbing olive oil around the edge of the garlic to decrease skin irritation. Cover with a bandage and leave in place for at least a few hours.

PLANT·GROW·HARVEST·USE

When I'm feeling weary (all that weeding, after all), I consider becoming a garlic grower, because compared to so many other vegetables, fruits, and herbs, it's extremely easy to grow, and does well in a range of conditions.

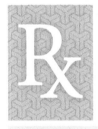

MEDICINE CABINET

Garlic's potency is derived from active compounds that include allyl sulfur, which is converted to allicilin when a clove is chopped and *allowed to stand for fifteen minutes*. Allicilin is anti-fungal, anti-bacterial, anti-viral, and anti-inflammatory. But it's pro-delicious.

Significant anti-bacterial activity

Scientific research supports many of garlic's traditional uses. Researchers reported that garlic exhibited anti-bacterial activity against gram positive (*Bacillu subtilis, Staphylococcus aureu*) and gram negative (*Escherichia coli* and *Klebsiella pneumonia*) strains and anti-fungal activity against *Candida albicans*.[1]

Reduces inflammation

Researchers noted that aged garlic extract plus CoQ10 greatly reduced inflammatory markers and reduced progression of coronary atherosclerosis.[2]

1. B Meriga et al., "Insecticidal, Antimicrobial and Antioxidant Activities of Bulb Extracts of Allium Sativum," *Asian Pacific Journal of Tropical Medicine* May 2012: 391-395. http://www.ncbi.nlm.nih.gov/pubmed/22546657.

2. Zeb, I., et al. "Aged Garlic Extract and Coenzyme Q10 Have Favorable Effect on Inflammatory Markers and Coronary Atherosclerosis Progression: A Randomized Clinical Trial," *Journal of Cardiovascular Disease Research* 2012 July; 185-190. http://www.ncbi.nlm.nih.gov/pubmed/22923934

CHECKLIST

Sun: Six to eight hours per day

Shade: Full sun to partial shade

Soil: Well-drained, loosened soil

Fertilizer: Not necessary, but does need mulch to retain moisture

Pests: Tend to be minimal; can be subject to viruses

Water: Occasionally, depending on soil dryness

Grow Indoors? No

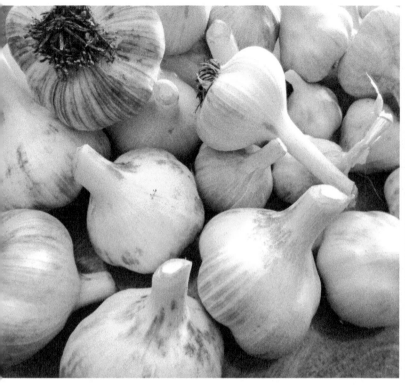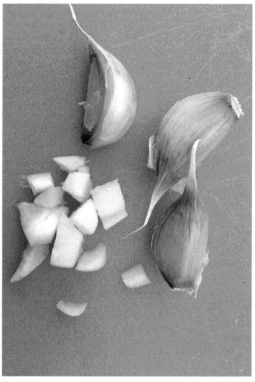

VARIETIES Garlic has two main categories: softneck, which does best in warmer climates where winter is mild, and hardneck, a good choice for climates where winter sees plummeting temperatures. Within those, there is an array of options when it comes to varieties:

- **Inchelium Red:** A softneck that hails from Washington state. It has a pleasant, mild taste, and a good growing history.
- **Nootka Rose:** Also a softneck, this variety tends to have strong leaves and stems, which makes it nice if you want to braid the garlic stems.
- **Chesnok Red:** This variety is part of a hardneck category called "purple stripe," named for its streaks of purplish color just under the thin white wrappers. Very pretty, with bold flavor.
- **French Rocambole:** Another category of hardnecks is Rocambole, known for rounded bulbs and strong garlic flavor. They also feature looser wrappers, which makes them easier to peel.
- **Georgian Crystal:** Part of the Porcelain category of hardnecks, this produces large cloves with reddish brown skin.

PLANT It's possible to plant garlic from seed, but not many growers attempt it. Instead, purchase seed garlic, which are bulbs grown specifically for propagation. Although you could take a garlic bulb from the grocery store and plant its cloves, that's inadvisable because the variety may not be suitable for your particular climate, and sometimes those bulbs have been sprayed to prevent sprouting—the very thing you need the cloves to do.

Because garlic needs at least two months of 40-degree temperatures to produce bulbs, it's best to plant in the fall and then overwinter the garlic so it germinates fully in the spring. If you miss your fall window, give it a shot in the spring. Most likely, they'll still germinate and mature, but your bulbs could be smaller than those that overwintered.

To plant, break the bulb into individual cloves, and use the largest cloves. (You can plant the tiny ones, but you'll likely harvest very small bulbs.) One end will be flatter, and the other end pointed—plant so that the pointed end is up. Dig a small trench about 2 to 3 inches deep and place garlic 6 to 8 inches apart. Cover, and then mulch the bed with at least a few inches of straw to protect the small shoots from freezing.

On our farm, we avoid fungal and viral issues by first soaking the garlic in a mixture of seaweed and vodka for about ten minutes before planting. The result is healthy, abundant garlic, and plenty of jokes about drinking a "garlictini."

GROW Here's the good news: garlic is very much a "set and forget" kind of plant. Once it's mulched, be sure to weed as needed, and pull the mulch back from around the garlic shoots in the spring so they don't get trapped under the hay or straw. Beyond that, you can leave it alone to work its magic.

HARVEST & STORE About a month before it's ready to harvest, garlic will develop a "scape" that curls up from the center. These are the flower stalks that, if left on, eventually form small bulbils that can be planted to grow more garlic, and also contain medicinal properties. Usually, they're cut off the plant so that energy doesn't get diverted from bulb formation. To cut the scape, clip as low as possible, right above the top leaf. The scapes can be chopped up and used in place of onions, and it imparts a mild garlic taste that's amazing. Many people make pesto, and we love to throw them on the grill after rubbing with olive oil, since the scape will crisp up.

When the garlic is ready the harvest, the lower leaves will turn a yellowish brown, with the top leaves still green. Gently use a pitchfork or garden tool to loosen the soil around the garlic, then pull it up, leaving the stalks on.

You can eat this fresh garlic, but it's better to cure the plant to prolong its storage capacity. Brush large bits of dirt from the bulb, but don't wash or clean too thoroughly, then hang the garlic or dry flat in a shady spot with good airflow. Farmers use a barn, but I've seen home gardeners utilize rafters on a porch, beams in a shed, or even basement spaces for hanging garlic (use a box fan to get some air circulation if this is your method). In about two weeks, the bulbs inside the wrappers will dry, and you can cut off the stalks and store the bulbs or use them. You can also save these bulbs for planting the next garlic round.

In terms of preparation, garlic can enhance just about any dish I can imagine, except perhaps cereal or cupcakes. Slice thin, for pasta sauces, or add chunky pieces to salsa, soups, stews, and other dishes.

NUTRITIONAL VALUE OF GARLIC

per 100 g (3.5 oz)

Garlic is rich in potassium and vitamin C.

Energy	149 kcal
Carbohydrates	33.06 g
Dietary fiber	2.1 g
Fat	0.50 g
Protein	6.36 g
Water	58.58 g
Vitamin A	0 µg
Thiamine	0.20 µg
Riboflavin	0.110 mg
Niacin	0.70 mg
Vitamin B$_6$	1.235 µg
Folate	3 µg
Choline	0 mg
Vitamin C	31.2 mg
Vitamin E	0.08 mg
Vitamin K	1.7 µg
Calcium	181 mg
Iron	1.70 mg
Magnesium	25 mg
Manganese	0 mg
Phosphorus	153 mg
Potassium	401 mg
Sodium	17 mg
Zinc	1.16 mg

Source: USDA Nutrient Database

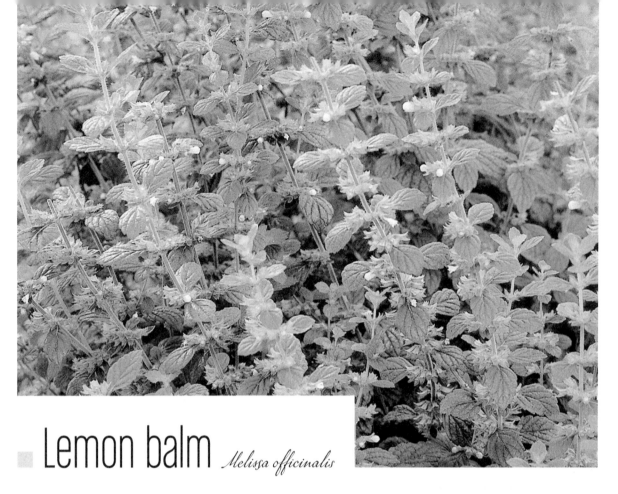

Lemon balm *Melissa officinalis*

Considered one of the cure-all types of herbs, lemon balm has a light citrus scent, especially when crushed, and is related to the mint family. During summer, small white flowers attract bees, giving the plant its botanical name (*Melissa* is Greek for "honeybee") and making an attractive complement to fruits, flowers, and vegetables that need pollinators. Thanks to its delicious flavor and stress-relieving benefits, lemon balm has long been used as a general health tonic and a flavoring added to candies and ice cream. In the 15th century, a Swiss physician dubbed it the "elixir of life," believing that regular use would raise the spirit and ensure continued wellness. In Austrian medicine, lemon balm leaves have regularly been used to treat the nervous system and gastrointestinal issues.

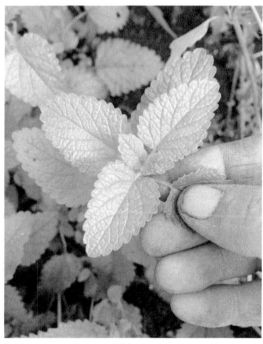

Lemon balm has hearty, thick leaves that are easy to harvest.

One of the herbal world's most calming options, lemon balm has also been known to settle the stomach, much like mint. It also boasts some antihistamine properties, helpful for combatting seasonal allergies.

Here are a few ideas for your Rx/medicinal preparations:

- For a chill-out tonic, create an infusion by pouring just-boiled water over 1 teaspoon dried or 2 teaspoons fresh lemon balm and letting steep for fifteen minutes. Cool, strain, and drink two to three times per day.
- Make a tincture as a digestive aid. Put 7 ounces dried or 14 ounces fresh into a liter of vodka and water and let steep for two weeks, shaking daily. Drink a small amount before meals.
- To repel mosquitoes, crush fresh leaves and rub on skin. Lemon balm contains the same properties as citronella, making it an excellent insect repellent.

CHECKLIST

Sun: Six to eight hours per day

Shade: Full sun or partial shade

Soil: Well-drained, loosened soil

Fertilizer: In spring and fall, followed by mulch

Pests: Tend to be minimal

Water: Regularly, depending on soil dryness

Grow Indoors? Yes

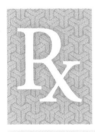

MEDICINE CABINET

One of the most promising aspects of lemon balm is its efficacy in treating children, as shown by numerous studies about restlessness and insomnia. Giving herbs to children makes many parents skittish—for good reason, as research is usually scant—so it's nice to have a go-to option that's well-tolerated in kids.

Effective for hyperactivity and concentration

Researchers examined whether lemon balm and valerian could be used for children suffering from hyperactivity and impulsiveness, ultimately improving concentration. They found significant improvement in the elementary school children studied who were given the herbs, leading them to conclude that lemon balm and valerian provide a viable option in addition to counseling and education.[1]

Helpful for sleep disorders during menopause

The onset of menopause is frequently associated with sleep disruption, with hot flashes intensifying insomnia, researchers noted. In attempting to find alternative therapies for the condition, researchers administered valerian and lemon balm to one group, and placebo to another. They found that "a significant difference was observed with reduced levels of sleep disorders amongst the experimental group when compared to the placebo group."[2]

1. Gromball, J. "Hyperactivity, concentration difficulties and impulsiveness improve during seven weeks' treatment with valerian root and lemon balm extracts in primary school children," *Phytomedicine* 2014 Jul-Aug; 21(8-9): 1098-103 http://www.ncbi.nlm.nih.gov/pubmed/24837472

2. Taavoni, S. "Valerian/lemon balm use for sleep disorders during menopause," *Complement Ther Clin Pract.* 2013 Nov; 19(4):193-6. http://www.ncbi.nlm.nih.gov/pubmed/24199972

PLANT·GROW·HARVEST·USE

Some herbs, like valerian or mullein, might require a hearty dose of motivation when using, since they're not exactly the tastiest options. But lemon balm is one of those delightfully good-smelling and great-tasting herbs that are easy to work into recipes and teas. Best of all, it's easy to grow and makes a nice addition to any ornamental landscape, thanks to its large, bright green leaves and late summer flowers.

VARIETIES The standard variety of lemon balm is called simply "common lemon balm," and is sold both as starter plants and as seeds. There are golden (called *aurea*) and variegated (called *variegata*) cultivars that exist, but they're not often offered through seed purveyors, and I've never seen them sold in any nurseries. That may be for good reason—those varieties tend to scorch with too much sun, making them a bit too fussy for home growers. Occasionally, it's possible to find different varieties like Lime, which boasts a lime scent and flavor, and Quedlinburger Niederliegende, which has a very high essential oil content, but it's more likely that you'll find common lemon balm over other varieties.

PLANT Lemon balm does well started indoors and then transplanted outside, so if you have a greenhouse space, that's ideal. However, even a kitchen windowsill will work. Place seeds in a tray or small individual pots, and water well. Once the plant is more established, transplant outdoors or into a large container, if that's where you plan to grow it. Or, transplant into a bigger pot for indoor growing so the roots have more room to expand.

Many gardeners buy transplants rather than starting from seed, and this can be a stellar jumpstart, especially since lemon balm is available at many nurseries and greenhouses. Look for hearty, well-established plants that have both established and new leaves. One advantage to buying transplants is that they've already been "hardened" (adapted) to outside temperatures, so they can be transplanted right away.

Aim for loose, well-drained soil in either outdoor or indoor planting. Lemon balm responds well to fertilization so work some organic nutrients into the soil, such as compost or blood meal.

If growing inside, make sure that the pot can drain properly—avoid letting the plant sit in water—so that the roots stay dry. If planting outside, be sure to loosen the soil around the transplant and avoid compaction when securing it in its new home.

Lemon balm in ice cubes makes a nice addition to lemonade.

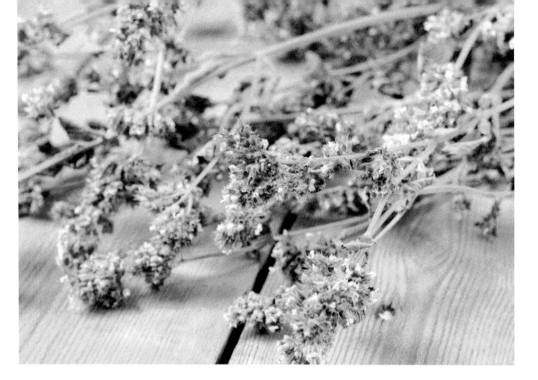

Lemon balm flowers are fragrant and edible, and dry well.

When the plant gets larger, add a layer of mulch around the roots so it can maintain adequate moisture levels, and doesn't have to compete with weeds.

GROW Although it's related to mint, lemon balm doesn't spread in the same way as that herb, but it *does* get bushy if it's not pruned regularly. To keep it from taking up too much space, cut lemon balm back often during the growing season, especially when it is flowering. Lemon balm seeds can spread throughout a garden, giving you more than you might need if you don't keep it under control.

To help manage it and to assist with root moisture, mulch in midsummer around the roots, which can help stop the spread of seeds and has the added benefit of creating more nutrients for the soil.

If the plant looks stressed, cut it back and it should rejuvenate with new growth. Also add some fertilizer, like compost, around the roots, especially if you've harvested numerous times.

HARVEST & STORE Although lemon balm flowers and stems can be harvested and dried, I've found the leaves to be the most flavorful and useful in terms of medicinal and culinary uses. They can be harvested anytime during the season, and the fresh leaves are delicious in teas and cocktails—try a few crushed leaves in a gin and tonic; it's a revelation.

Fresh leaves can also be substituted in place of mint in dishes, chopped into salads, and put into lemonade or water. Tearing the leaves helps to release the flavor, so I always do at least a quick crush or tear before using.

When the growing season starts winding down, dry the leaves on a clean mesh screen and crumble into an airtight glass jar, then store in a cool, dark cupboard. You can use the herb throughout the winter in teas and infusions, and they're especially helpful for the digestive system when you're eating heavy winter fare like roasts and stews. Keep in mind, though, that lemon balm loses a significant amount of its flavor when dried, so you may need to use much more for teas than you would have used fresh. But don't worry—soon enough, it'll be summer again.

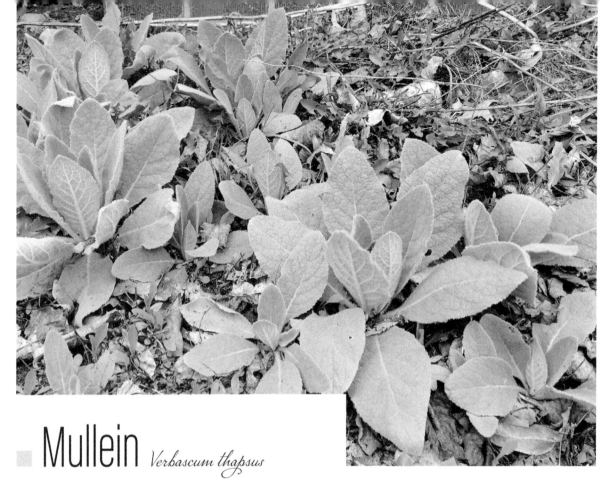

Mullein *Verbascum thapsus*

Herbs often have numerous other names and nicknames, but mullein might trump them all, with the designation of "grandmother's flannel" in reference to its soft, thick leaves. The wildflower often sprouts up in unexpected places (in the middle of a city sidewalk when I was an urban dweller, for example), and is remarkably tall, usually around 4 feet. The herb has been used for several purposes over the past few centuries, such as casting out evil spirits, and making wicks for candles since the leaves and stems ignite easily. In literature, Ulysses took mullein to protect himself against Circe, a goddess of magic. On the off chance that you don't have any spirits to dispel, and aren't on an epic journey worthy of literature, it can also be used to treat colds, sore throats, ear infections, and asthma.

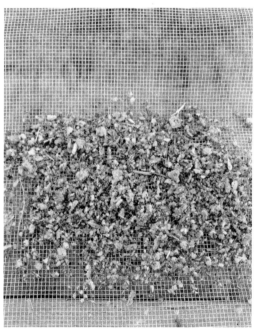

Mullein dries easily, and can then be chopped with a spice grinder.

Mullein has been smoked, burned as incense, and used for a wide range of medicinal applications, from pain management to respiratory issues.

Here are a few ideas for your Rx/medicinal preparations:

- For coughs, place fresh mullein leaves in a bowl and pour in boiling water; lean over the bowl with your head partially covered with a towel, for a steam inhalation that encourages respiratory cleansing.
- Create an ointment for chapped lips and skin by steeping flowers in olive oil for about three weeks in a glass jar; shake the jar every day to keep flowers from settling on the bottom.
- Staunch bleeding on minor wounds by snipping off a fresh leaf from the plant and holding against the wound until it stops bleeding.
- Dry leaves and flowers to make tea, which can act as a general tonic or work as a sedative or pain reliever.

PLANT·GROW·HARVEST·USE

Sometimes seen in abandoned lots and sidewalk cracks, mullein can become very sizeable, sometimes up to 8 feet tall, but usually stopping at about 4 feet. As its presence in poor soil indicates, the herb

CHECKLIST

Sun: Eight to ten hours per day

Shade: Full sun

Soil: Can thrive in poor soil

Fertilizer: Usually not necessary

Pests: Tend to be minimal

Water: Moderate watering

Grow Indoors? No

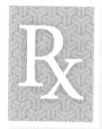

MEDICINE CABINET

Mullein has been found to kill viruses on contact, and a preliminary study suggests that the herb could help certain flu medications work better. The herb also contains saponins, which help to loosen mucus, which is why it's often recommended for issues like coughs and colds.

Antioxidant effect

Mullein has been used in European folk medicine due to its anti-inflammatory and soothing action on the respiratory tract, researchers noted. In a study of mullein extract, they also found that the herb contains polyphenols that play an important role in exerting an antioxidant effect on the body.[1]

Treatment for ear pain in children

Otitis media is one of the most frequent diseases of early infancy and childhood and one of the most common reasons that children visit a physician. In a study about naturopathic treatments, researchers found that mullein, along with other herbs such as lavender and calendula, can be beneficial in pain reduction in the condition.[2]

1. Grigore, A., "Correlation between polyphenol content and anti-inflammatory activity of Verbascum phlomoides (mullein)," *Pharm Biol* 2013 Jul; 51(7):925-9. http://www.ncbi.nlm.nih.gov/pubmed/23627472

2. Sarrell, E.M., "Naturopathic treatment for ear pain in children," *Pediatrics* 2003 May; 111(5 Pt 1):e574-9. http://www.ncbi.nlm.nih.gov/pubmed/12728112

thrives in disturbed and even contaminated soil, making it a strong choice for parts of your garden where other herbs have failed to grow, or where you'd like to enrich the soil for future planting.

VARIETIES When it comes to choices, mullein is very limited in variety. However, there are two main options that would do well in any garden, and are striking as ornamentals as well as medicinals:

- **Greek Mullein:** Because mullein flowers can be used in teas and tinctures, this variety will be especially prized by anyone who appreciates those flavors. Native to Greece, the variety boasts a wealth of upright yellow flowers that are easily stripped down for harvest.
- **Common Mullein:** Considered the most productive variety for leaf production; boasts thick, fuzzy leaves that are strong enough to be dried using a dehydrator.

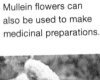

Mullein flowers can also be used to make medicinal preparations.

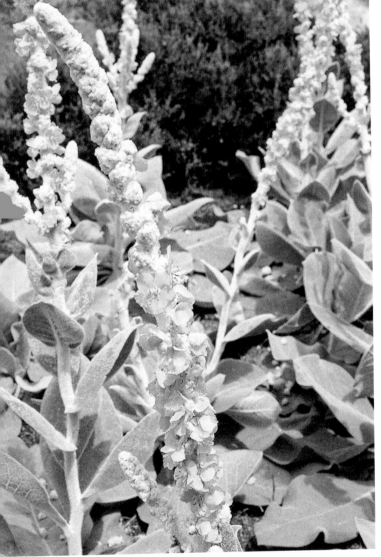

PLANT Because mullein is often found in vacant lots and is often considered a weed, I deliberated over whether to include it in the "Wild Yard Friends" section instead of cultivated medicinal herbs. Mullein did, in fact, create a constellation of fuzzy leaves along the lawn of my former house in Minneapolis, causing my fussy neighbor to issue all kinds of passive-aggressive comments about weed control.

Fortunately, I moved. And I began growing mullein instead of searching for it, and found that cultivation naturally required a different mindset and strategy than foraging. Another advantage to growing it deliberately is that you won't risk confusing mullein with foxglove, a plant that looks very similar and also has fuzzy leaves, but is considered toxic.

To grow mullein, it's best to plant seeds indoors in early spring—the seeds need light in order to germinate, and so would be too exposed to birds if planted outside. Instead, place seeds in small pots into potting soil and press slightly, then cover with a very thin layer of vermiculite, a silicate that promotes rapid root growth, anchors young roots, and helps with moisture retention.. In the case of mullein, it helps to let light in for the seeds, but still protects the top layer of the soil during the germination process.

You'll need that protection, because a thirty-day cold stratification process is recommended. That means mimicking the winter conditions necessary for a plant to emerge from winter's cooler temps. Cover the small pots with plastic wrap to retain moisture, and place in a refrigerator kept under 60 degrees Fahrenheit. The seeds should germinate in about two weeks, and then you can remove them and let them continue growing in room temperature. Once the plant has two leaves, you can transplant them outdoors.

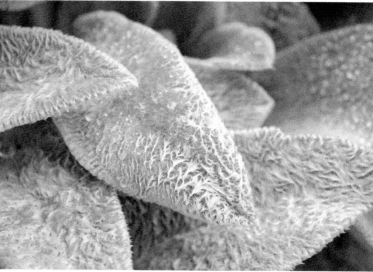

The leaves on mullein can be thick and almost furry.

GROW Once mullein begins to establish, it grows well without much maintenance. This is a plant that can grow as tall as a basketball player, after all, in the middle of an empty parking lot. However, if you're in the midst of drought-type conditions, water whenever the soil seems especially dry. Also, trim dead leaves from the bottom in order to encourage more growth.

Mullein is one of the few biennial herbs, which means it takes two years to mature. The first season, you'll get only a small plant of downy leaves, looking like a rosette frosting accent on a cake. But the next summer, you'll get the long flowering stalk that delivers the most medicinal clout. If your garden tends to be windy, considering staking the plant in its second year so it can maintain height.

HARVEST & STORE If you're planning to use a variety that flowers abundantly, like Greek mullein, flower harvesting takes only moments—just grasp the bottom of a flower stem and zip your fingers upward while holding a bag or bowl underneath. This differs from common mullein, which is harvested by picking flowers individually.

Dry the flowers on a clean mesh screen, and either store in an airtight glass jar or use immediately to make a tea or tincture. Similarly, pick the fuzzy leaves, typically after the morning dew has burned off, and lay on the screen for drying as well. Because the leaves are so thick and hearty, they can also be dried in a dehydrator, on the lowest setting.

You can harvest leaves during the first year of growing, while flowers can be collected from two-year-old plants. Important note: don't eat mullein seeds, since they can be irritating to the system, but you can use the seeds to propagate mullein in other parts of a garden.

One last and very odd use: mullein for fishing. Anyone who's read *Love in the Time of Cholera* by Gabriel Garcia Marquez might remember a scene where characters put mullein in the water as they were fishing. Because the herb contains saponins, a compound that's toxic to insects and fish—but harmless to people—throwing mullein in the water stuns the fish and causes them to float onto the water's surface, where they're easily scooped up. In Marquez's scene, the practice is so effective that "the sea seemed paved with aluminum."

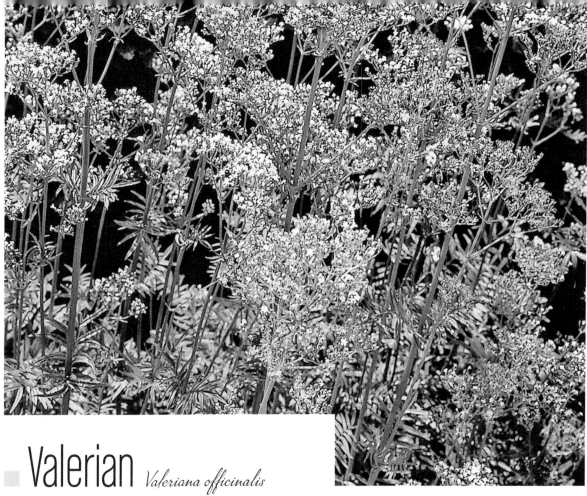

Valerian *Valeriana officinalis*

One of the best-known herbal sedatives, valerian was used during both World War I and World War II to treat battle-related stress. Before that, the perennial flowering plant was used to make perfume extracts in the 16th century, and was favored in ancient Greece for treating ailments of the urinary tract, liver, and digestive system. Valerian was once used as a spice, and its roots added to stews or softened enough to be added to salads. Although it's not consumed much (if ever) in the US as an edible, the herb continues to be added to dishes in other parts of the world. In addition to medicinal and culinary uses, valerian was once thought to bring squabbling couples back together, and acted as a major ingredient in love spells.

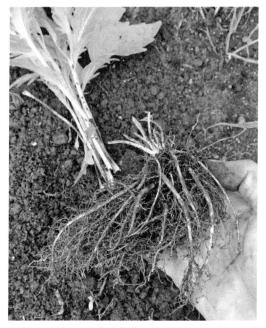

Valerian root is somewhat shallow, so it's easy to dig up.

Valerian is the ultimate chill-out herb, and has been noted as one of the most effective plants for lowering blood pressure. As with many herbs, valerian shouldn't be taken indefinitely; instead, use for a couple weeks, then take a week off from the herb before resuming use.

Here are a few ideas for your Rx/medicinal preparations:

* For a general calming effect, make a tonic wine by using about 2 ounces of the dried root; crush and add to 1 cup of dry white wine, then steep for a month, gently shaking occasionally. Use up to three times daily or as needed.

* To relieve PMS symptoms or assist with insomnia, create an infusion by crushing a teaspoon of fresh valerian root and soaking in a cup of room-temperature water for at least twelve hours. Strain, and then drink a small cup in the evening.

* To create a compress for drawing out a splinter or bee stinger, make the infusion double strength and soak a clean cloth in the liquid, and then apply to the affected area.

CHECKLIST

Sun: Six to eight hours per day

Shade: Full sun to partial shade

Soil: Well-drained, loosened soil

Fertilizer: Compost and mulch in spring and autumn

Pests: Tend to be minimal

Water: Keep area moist but not soaked

Grow Indoors? Yes

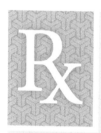

MEDICINE CABINET

Considered an effective stress reliever, valerian has often been studied along with other calmative herbs like chamomile, lemon balm, and evening primrose as methods for addressing insomnia, anxiety, and depression.

Effective for hyperactivity and concentration

Researchers examined whether lemon balm and valerian could be used for children suffering from hyperactivity and impulsiveness, ultimately improving concentration. They found significant improvement in the elementary school children studied who were given the herbs, leading them to conclude that lemon balm and valerian provide a viable option in addition to counseling and education.[1]

Helpful for sleep disorders during menopause

The onset of menopause is frequently associated with sleep disruption, with hot flashes intensifying insomnia, researchers noted. In attempting to find alternative therapies for the condition, researchers administered valerian and lemon balm to one group, and placebo to another. They found that "a significant difference was observed with reduced levels of sleep disorders amongst the experimental group when compared to the placebo group."[2]

1. Gromball, J. "Hyperactivity, concentration difficulties and impulsiveness improve during seven weeks' treatment with valerian root and lemon balm extracts in primary school children," *Phytomedicine* 2014 Jul-Aug; 21(8-9): 1098-103 http://www.ncbi.nlm.nih.gov/pubmed/24837472

2. Taavoni, S. "Valerian/lemon balm use for sleep disorders during menopause," *Complement Ther Clin Pract.* 2013 Nov; 19(4):193-6. http://www.ncbi.nlm.nih.gov/pubmed/24199972

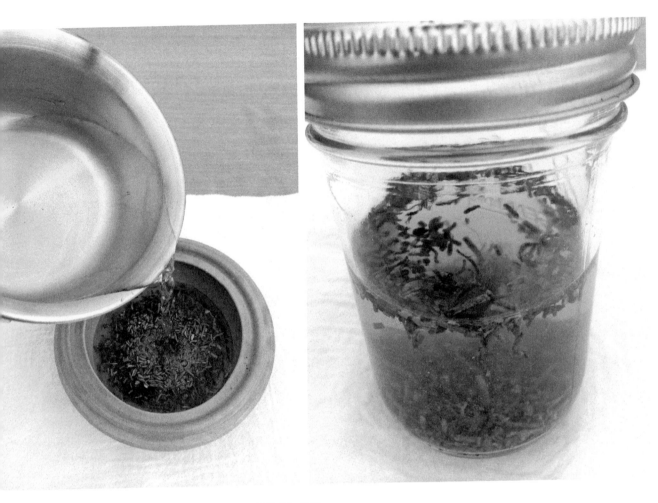

Left: To make a preparation, first pour boiling water over the roots.

Right: Valerian leaves can also be used and made into a tea.

PLANT·GROW·HARVEST·USE

A towering perennial, valerian can grow to about 5 feet tall and often sports white flowers that provide a happy space for bees and butterflies. Because of that, it's advisable to plant near vegetables and fruits that can benefit from pollinators, such as melons, tomatoes, or cucumbers. Its robust size also makes a nice backdrop to an ornamental landscape, and it trellises well on fencing.

VARIETIES The standard variety of valerian is called simply "common valerian," or "official valerian" in reference to its botanical name. This type is native to Europe and temperate parts of Asia, and is remarkably hardy, down to -20 degrees Fahrenheit. Although other varieties are sometimes mentioned, finding seeds for these is difficult, and it's much easier to secure the familiar, well-known variety.

PLANT Although valerian can be grown from seed, germination can be tricky, so it's best grown through root division. Dig up a small amount of an existing plant, leaving the majority of the roots in place, and transplant into a your garden space after loosening the soil. Place transplants into the soil carefully, and water thoroughly to help reduce shock. Mulch around the roots to assist with moisture control.

If you prefer to give seeding a try, start the seeds indoors in a small container (about 2 inches or so) first, which will keep the roots warmer, aiding in germination. Cover with a very thin layer of vermiculite, a silicate that's fluffy and pebble-shaped. It helps to promote fast root growth, anchor young roots, boost moisture retention, and assist germination. Look for horticultural vermiculite, as opposed to other types that are used for shipping chemicals or enriching concrete. In the case of valerian, it helps to let light in for the seeds, but still protects the top layer of the soil during the germination process.

As the plant grows larger, transfer to a larger container (at least 6 inches deep) so the roots can establish more firmly. Transplant outside in early spring, after the last frost.

Use valerian seeds as soon as you can; they don't store for long and germination suffers if you're using seeds that are left over from the previous season.

GROW Once valerian is established, maintenance is minimal. It's best to mulch around the roots each spring and autumn so that roots are well protected.

Keep in mind that cats *love* valerian, usually as much as catnip, and some ancient herbalists would gauge a plant's potency based on how eager cats were to destroy it. If kitties are becoming an issue, consider some fencing or netting, but in general, if your cats are rolling in the valerian, it means you have a good crop.

HARVEST & STORE Although valerian leaves can be dried and used, the part of the plant most commonly used is its potent roots. Wait till after the plant's flowering and summer stages and harvest part of the roots in late autumn of its second year, once the greens have died back and the plant's energy is going into the roots to prepare for winter. Be sure to leave enough roots to keep the plant healthy for the next season—that's not too difficult since even a small amount of the roots can be potent, and it only takes about a teaspoon of ground roots to make an infusion.

During the autumn, you can use fresh roots, as long as they're thoroughly washed and allowed to dry. For preparations during the winter, let the roots dry in a well-ventilated area and store in an airtight glass jar in a cool, dark place.

One important note: valerian root has a very distinct aroma, which I tend to equate with dirty feet. Be prepared. If the smell bothers you too much while drinking tea, you can also get valerian's benefits by putting some powdered root into empty gelatin capsules, available at co-ops, online, or some drug stores.

You can also dry the leaves to use as a tea for relaxation and insomnia. They aren't as potent as the root, but they're also much less stinky.

NUTRITIONAL VALUE OF VALERIAN

The nutritional value of valerian has not been established.

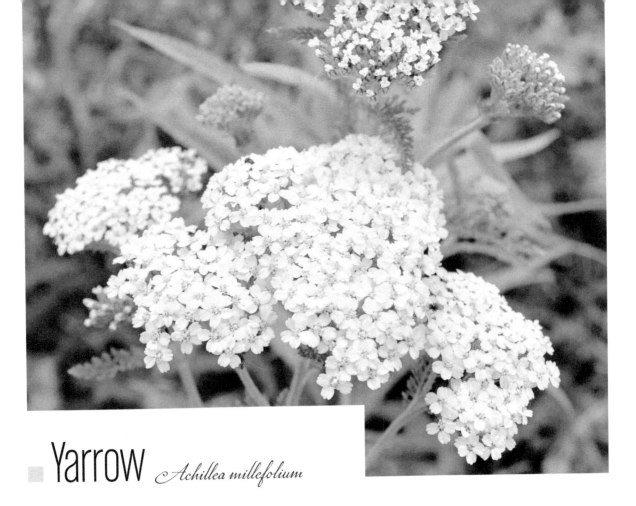

Yarrow *Achillea millefolium*

As seen in its botanical genus name, yarrow was reportedly named after Greek hero Achilles, who used the herb to help his soldiers stop bleeding (apparently it doesn't work as well on the vulnerable heels of mythical Greek heroes). Since then, the herb has been common in European herbal remedies, in part because yarrow contains flavonoids, a compound that increases stomach acid and saliva and helps with digestion. In general, though, the herb is best known for its ability to staunch wounds and stop bleeding, and some herbal practitioners recommend chewing the fresh herb briefly—which creates an added benefit of helping internal maladies—and placing the resulting mash onto open wounds. If you can get the son of a Greek god to do this for you, then by all means, pursue that route.

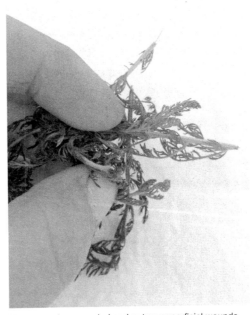

Yarrow can be crumpled and put on superficial wounds.

Often used as a garden ornamental, yarrow is a standout when it comes to medicinal purposes. The flowering tops are used to stop bleeding, and can be taken internally as a tonic for uterine health and gastrointestinal wellness.

Here are a few ideas for your Rx/medicinal preparations:

- When you've experienced a small wound or gash, chew a few leaves of yarrow until it's a mushy mass. Place on the wound in a poultice fashion, and wrap fresh, clean gauze over the chewed yarrow to stop bleeding. Avoid using on any deep cuts, since these should be treated medically instead.
- Create an infusion by pouring just-boiled water over fresh or dried yarrow flowers; use to induce sweating after a fever as a way to detoxify the body.
- Make a yarrow tonic wine by putting 3 ounces of fresh or dry flowers in 1 liter of white wine for thirty days. Strain, and drink a tablespoon daily to help absorb nutrients from meals.

PLANT·GROW·HARVEST·USE

As a perennial, yarrow has wide flower heads that are comprised of numerous, tightly packed flowers. The leaves resemble ferns, and have a delicate, wispy look when the plant is just establishing. Because of the herb's pretty look and aromatic leaves, it makes a nice ornamental choice, particularly if you're going for a "wildflower" kind of landscape.

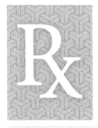

MEDICINE CABINET

The young leaves of yarrow can be eaten fresh, and some people chew the leaves to relieve toothaches or to address gum issues. Herbalists have also recommended the herb for colds, loss of appetite, and gastrointestinal complaints. Unfortunately, the herb hasn't been formally studied much, but hopefully, researchers will pick up on its benefits soon.

Addresses severe colds

Yarrow tea can help severe colds, especially those that result in fever and obstructed perspiration, herbalists note. An infusion made with a little cayenne pepper helps to open the pores and purify the blood.[1]

Long medicinal history

Yarrow has a rich history of being used as a medicinal treatment, since before the Bronze Age, according to a noted herbalist. The herb has been known for thousands of years as a treatment for wounds, and imparts antiseptic qualities that help staunch bleeding.[2]

1. http://www.botanical.com/botanical/mgmh/y/yarrow02.html#med
2. http://www.ryandrum.com/threeherbs.htm

CHECKLIST

Sun: Six to eight hours per day

Shade: Full sun

Soil: Well-drained, loosened soil

Fertilizer: A layer of compost under mulch when planting

Pests: Tend to be minimal

Water: When soil seems dry

Grow Indoors? No

VARIETIES When choosing a yarrow variety, you'll usually be making a choice based on color. At our farm, we've found that white yarrow grows best, germinates more reliably, and is considered the most medicinally active variety. But I've spoken to others who prefer other flower colors because they add more interest in a garden mix. Here are a few other options:

- **Coastal:** Native to the coasts of Oregon and California, this temperate-climate yarrow has the largest flower head, and is extremely aromatic, making it especially tempting to pollinators.
- **Colorado Mix:** Huge flower heads in multiple colors make this variety a stunner. The colors range from red, pink, yellow, and apricot, and flowers have a long life when cut for bouquets.
- **Cloth of Gold:** This variety would be better named "cloth of butter" since the hue is a bright, fresh yellow.
- **Parker's Variety:** A hardy yarrow with feathery gray-green foliage and tiny yellow flowers.

PLANT Yarrow can be direct-seeded into a garden, but establishes better if it's transplanted from a start that's been nurtured indoors for about six to eight weeks before transplanting outside. If you want to speed germination, cover the top of a seeded pot with plastic wrap, which will trap moisture and heat inside, and remove the wrap when the seeds have sprouted.

You can also find yarrow, on occasion, at greenhouses and nurseries as an established start, and this is always a nice option if you're running out of transplant space inside (believe me, I know the feeling).

Before transplanting outside, pick a spot with full sunshine and soil that drains well. Compacted soil will result in slow growth, or even no growth at all, so if your chosen yarrow spot seems dense, loosen up the area with a pitchfork or other cultivating tool. Although it sounds counterintuitive, consider a spot where other herbs have struggled or failed in the past. Yarrow does well with average-to-poor soil, although it can thrive in rich soil as well.

When planting, space plants 1 to 2 feet apart, since some varieties can grow up to 4 feet tall.

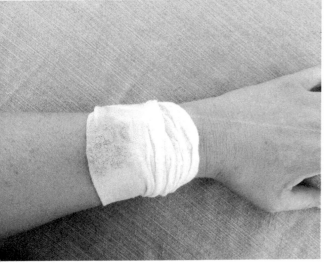

A yarrow poultice can be helpful to stop bleeding.

Once the herb begins to establish, add a thin layer of compost (non-manure kind) followed by a few inches of mulch to help keep the roots moist but not wet.

GROW Most likely, you'll just be paying attention to yarrow during harvest, or whenever there are drought conditions that require some occasional watering. Otherwise, the herb thrives on its own.

Because yarrow is a perennial and will come back each spring, prepare for the season by adding a new layer of compost and a thin layer of mulch each spring, and clearing away any debris or weeds from the previous season.

This herb does well if you thin it occasionally, making sure to give new growth plenty of room to spread out. Fortunately, you don't need to compost what you've thinned if you're

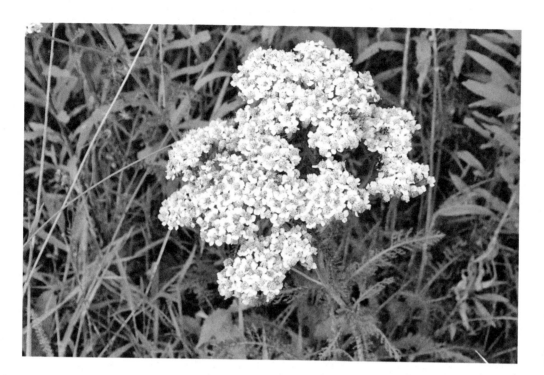

Yarrow is easy to spot in the wild, thanks to the umbrella-like shape of its blooms.

NUTRITIONAL VALUE OF YARROW

The nutritional value of yarrow has not been established.

removing healthy plants as you thin them; simply replant what's been divided out in well-prepared soil someplace else in the garden. This might be a good time to offer yarrow to your neighbors, creating an area that's ideal for beneficial insects and will attract happy bees.

HARVEST & STORE Yarrow flowers and leaves are the most utilized, although you can also use the stems if you don't feel like removing them before putting other dried components in a spice grinder.

Harvest when the plant is in full flower, and dry the flowers and leaves on a clean mesh, then crumble or grind and store in an airtight glass jar in a cool, dark location. You can use the dried flowers to make a tincture by using about ½-teaspoon dried yarrow to 1 cup just-boiled water, and letting it steep for about five minutes. After straining, the tincture can be used as a tea, or made into a wound cleanser to control bleeding.

In the fall, harvest part of the yarrow root, but instead of drying it as you would with other herb roots, chew while it's still fresh to relieve tooth pain.

Keep in mind that when using yarrow, particularly as a tea, you'll likely work up a sweat. That's because yarrow tends to raise body heat, and flush infection and fever out. That's excellent for detox purposes, but you may not want to be sipping yarrow tea during an important work meeting, for example.

One important note about interactions: medications that slow blood clotting can interact negatively with yarrow. These drugs include some prescription meds like heparin and warfarin, but also common over-the-counter choices like aspirin, ibuprofen, and naproxen. So, if you're taking one of those, skip the yarrow until you're off that medication.

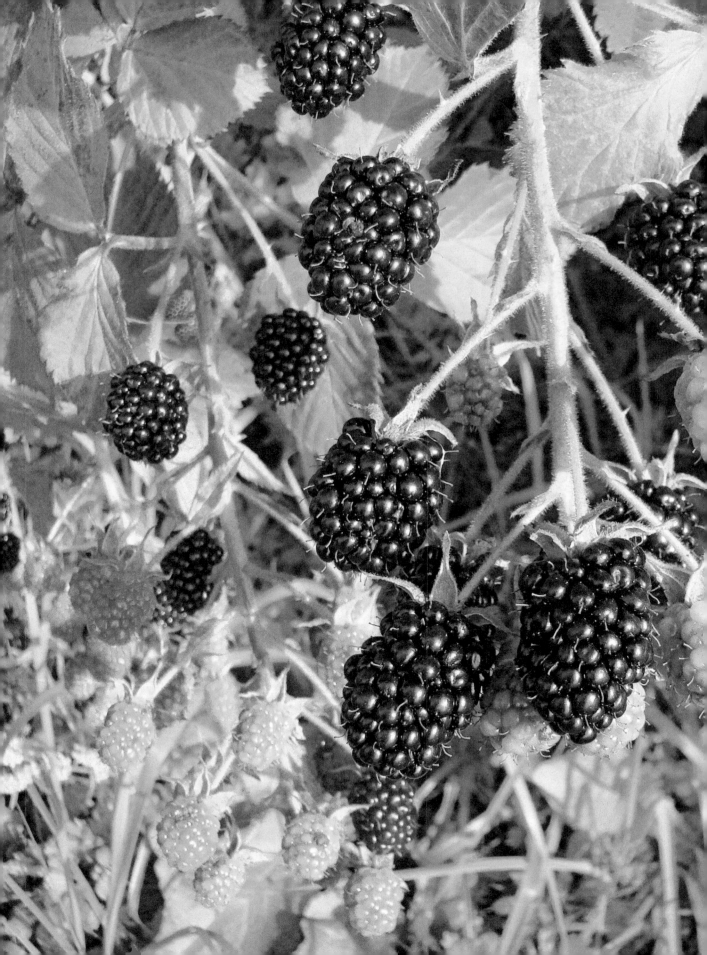

FIVE

Fruits and Shrubs

While nearly all of the previous chapters focused on herbs, throwing a few edibles into the mix makes sense in terms of wellness. Of course vegetables are packed with vitamins, minerals, and other goodness, and it's much easier to grill an onion than a sprig of basil. Fruits, on the other hand, tend to get less attention. So, let's change that.

Although fruits are well recognized for their antioxidant power and sweetness, they're not often heralded for the incredible amount of medicinal clout that they can bring. Dried or fresh, selections like blackberry, blueberry, and strawberry are more than a natural way to lighten up your morning granola, or to bake into a sugar-drenched pie.

Best of all, fruits make a fantastic addition to any backyard pharmacy because they're generally easy to plant and maintain, and offer fruits year after year. You can create an espalier by trellising them along a wall, or keep shrubs nestled alongside a walkway for a more ornamental effect. Creating a space for fruit plants might be as simple as utilizing a vacant stretch next to a fence, or covering the back of the garage with vines and bushes.

As long as you can control the birds, squirrels, and neighbor children, it's likely you'll have bountiful harvests for years to come. When it comes to wellness (and deliciousness), give fruits a chance.

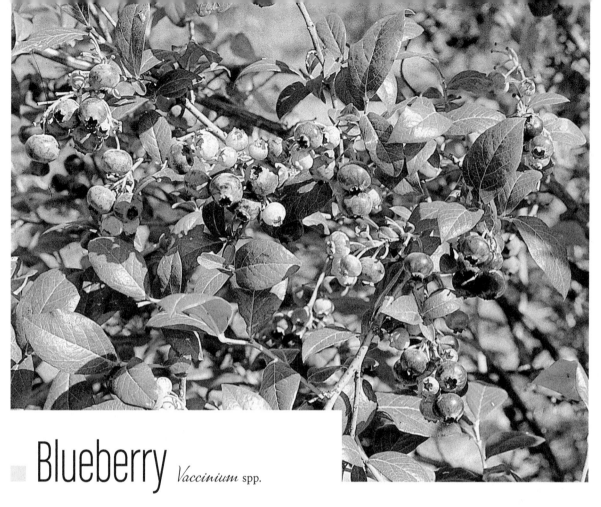

Blueberry *Vaccinium* spp.

Unlike many types of herbs and fruits which were introduced into the United States and Canada from other parts of the world, the blueberry is native to North America and is now grown commercially in South America, Australia, New Zealand, and parts of Europe. Here's a fun fact for my fellow berry geeks: Georgia has become one of the biggest producers in the global blueberry market, since it has such a long harvest season, from April to August. (Take that, peaches.) But Maine produces a significant amount of lowbush/wild blueberries, and there's a town in New Jersey that calls itself the "Blueberry Capital of the World." It's a daring boast, Hammonton, N.J., but we admire your boldness. Another trivia moment: blueberries are Canada's largest fruit crop. Medicinally, the fruit is a powerhouse antioxidant, helping to treat everything from digestive issues to eyesight problems.

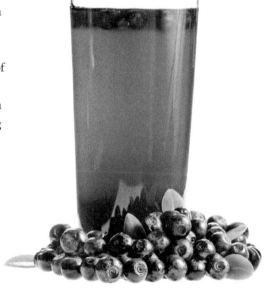

Blueberry tea is a delicious and medicinal summer drink.

Blueberries have been used medicinally for centuries, particularly by Native American peoples. Blueberry juice has been noted for its beneficial effects on the urinary tract, helping to lower inflammation and inhibit the growth of certain bacteria. Best of all, the berries and their leaves are simple to use for better health.

Here are a few ideas for your Rx/medicinal preparations:

- For treatment of diarrhea, create a tincture by macerating some dried blueberries in alcohol for a week to ten days, then putting about twenty to thirty drops in a glass of water. Drink twice per day until there's digestive relief. This remedy is also useful for indigestion, bloating, or gas.
- Snack on them. All the antioxidant properties will be present, plus fiber, and of course, that super fresh *pop* of flavor with every bite.
- Dry the blueberry leaves and make into a tea as a general health tonic, or to help with issues related to the urinary tract, eye health, or digestive system.

PLANT·GROW·HARVEST·USE

When considering blueberry plants for your home garden, there are a few definitions that should be kept in mind, since you'll encounter them when choosing plants:

CHECKLIST

Sun: Eight to ten hours per day

Shade: Full sun

Soil: Well-drained, loosened soil

Fertilizer: Use if plant seems to be struggling

Pests: Tend to be minimal, but look out for viruses

Water: Regularly, depending on soil dryness

Grow Indoors? No

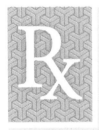

MEDICINE CABINET

Blueberries are one of the shining stars of the antioxidant universe, and they've been touted for medicinal uses that range from easing gout symptoms to boosting urinary health.

Promising for issues in older adults

Researchers have noted that the prevalence of dementia is increasing with the expansion of an older adult population. One study has found that daily consumption of blueberry juice led to improved memory, reduced depressive symptoms, and lower glucose levels.[1]

Potential role in prevention of cancer and vascular diseases

A study in *Molecular Nutrition & Food Research* suggests that blueberries and cranberries could have the ability to "limit the development and severity of certain cancers and vascular diseases including atherosclerosis, ischemic stroke and neurodegenerative diseases of aging," thanks to a variety of phytochemicals.[2]

1. Krikorian, R., et al. "Blueberry supplementation improves memory in older adults," *Journal of Agricultural and Food Chemistry* 2010 Apr; 58(7): 3996-4000. http://www.ncbi.nlm.nih.gov/pubmed/20047325

2. Neto, C. "Cranberry and blueberry: Evidence for protective effects against cancer and vascular diseases," *Molecular Nutrition & Food Research* 2007 June; 6:652-664. http://onlinelibrary.wiley.com/doi/10.1002/mnfr.200600279/abstract

- **Highbush:** This is a type of cultivated blueberry plant that does well in cooler climates, such as Zone 6 or cooler (lower zone numbers).
- **Rabbiteye:** This cultivated plant is geared toward more temperate areas like Zone 7 and warmer (higher zone numbers). It's sometimes referred to as southern highbush.
- **Lowbush:** This term is used often for wild blueberries, which produce smaller berries than highbush or rabbiteye, but there are many lowbush varieties that can be cultivated. These are creeper plants, only about a foot high.

Keep in mind that these aren't varieties (those are in the next section), but *categories* of blueberry plants. Sometimes, when people have trouble growing blueberries, they've chosen plants that don't work well for their climate.

VARIETIES Much like blackberries, blueberry plants can be chosen based on when they fruit—early season, midseason, late midseason, and late season. Some people plant several varieties so they can have blueberries for months. (Those people are called geniuses.) There are dozens of blueberry varieties, with these as a small sampling:

- **Patriot:** If you're in a colder climate with a shorter growing season, this is a good variety; developed by the University of Maine, it's also particularly winter hardy.
- **Bluecrop:** A popular commercial variety with high yields and large firm berries.
- **Chandler:** Considered the largest berry variety, and well suited for Zones 5 to 7 but it's not hardy enough for cooler areas.
- **Jersey:** One of the oldest and most widely grown varieties, with high yields and late-season berries. Since it has a nice shape, it tends to be a good ornamental variety too.

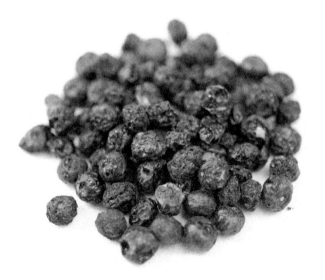

Dried blueberries are easy to store for long periods of time.

PLANT Like other berry types, blueberries prefer full sun, and will grow in partial shade, but fruit production could be lower in those areas. The most important consideration when planting will be the soil—blueberries thrive best with soil that's rich with organic matter, drains well, and has a lower pH (more acidic). The proper blueberry soil pH level is between 4 and 5, which tends to be lower than most garden soils. To drop pH levels, add granular sulfur to the soil (math moment: about 1 pound of sulfur per 50 feet will lower the pH by one point). Work it well into the soil, ideally at least a few months before planting.

If you happen to be friends with your local coffee shop owner, skip the sulfur and topdress with used coffee grounds instead. You'll need *plenty*, probably about 4 to 6 inches worth above the soil, but it's a nice way to acidify the soil.

Once the soil is ready, plant in early spring, and space bushes about 5 feet apart. Water well to get the plants established, and fertilize about a month after planting rather than at planting time.

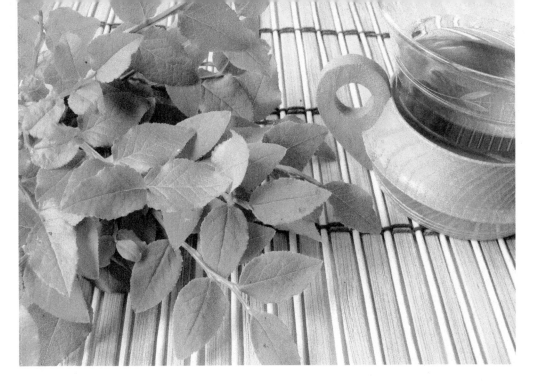

Blueberry leaves can be dried and made into tea.

NUTRITIONAL VALUE OF BLUEBERRIES

per 100 g (3.5 oz)

Blueberries are rich in vitamin K, manganese, vitamin C, and fiber.

Energy	57 kcal
Carbohydrates	14.49 g
Dietary fiber	2.4 g
Fat	.33 g
Protein	0.74 g
Water	84.21 g
Vitamin A	3 µg
Thiamine	0.0513 µg
Riboflavin	0.041 mg
Niacin	0.418 mg
Vitamin B$_6$	0.052 µg
Folate	6 µg
Choline	0 mg
Vitamin C	9.7 mg
Vitamin E	0.57 mg
Vitamin K	19.3 µg
Calcium	6 mg
Iron	0.28 mg
Magnesium	6 mg
Protein	0.74 mg
Phosphorus	12 mg
Potassium	77 mg
Sodium	1 mg
Zinc	0.16 mg
Sodium	17 mg
Zinc	1.16 mg

Source: USDA Nutrient Database

GROW Blueberries have shallow root systems, so they do well with mulching since it keeps the roots moist. Apply a layer of hay, wood chips, leaves, pine needs or other mulch after planting.

Although some varieties will produce fruit during the first year, I've heard a number of gardening experts recommend prevention of fruit production until a couple years after planting. Believe me, it breaks my heart, but it really does work to create a stronger, more productive plant for the future. Just pinch back the blossoms when you see them, and think about the value of long-term gain versus short-term blueberry cobblers.

One more important note: birds. Wow, do they ever love blueberries! Try some netting over the plants as a deterrent, and offer some suet cakes nearby to distract them.

HARVEST & STORE Harvesting blueberries is one of those bucolic, dreamy moments that showcase the feeling of summer. Think that's hyperbole? Then grab a bucket, stand in front of a blueberry bush, and try not to sigh with happiness as you pluck, pluck, sample, and pluck.

In the heart of summer, I try to eat as many fresh blueberries as possible, although I do put some in our food dehydrator to preserve for granola and other dishes in the winter. Also, some studies have found that freezing blueberries doesn't damage their antioxidant levels, so if I can't get fresh or don't have the time to dry them, I freeze as many as I can get. Fortunately, cooking doesn't result in significant loss of antioxidants, so that's another option.

To freeze blueberries properly, line a small cookie sheet (which needs to fit in your freezer) with wax paper and put the blueberries on it in a single layer. Freeze overnight, then break up any clumped-together berries; put all into a plastic freezer bag. This method will keep the blueberries from forming into a solid mass, which would happen if you skipped the initial freezing step.

The blueberry leaves can also be used for teas and tinctures, so pick them just before the fruit appears, when the leaves are at full potency, and dry them on a clean mesh screen away from drafts. When dried, pack into a glass jar, seal tightly, and store in a cool, dark place.

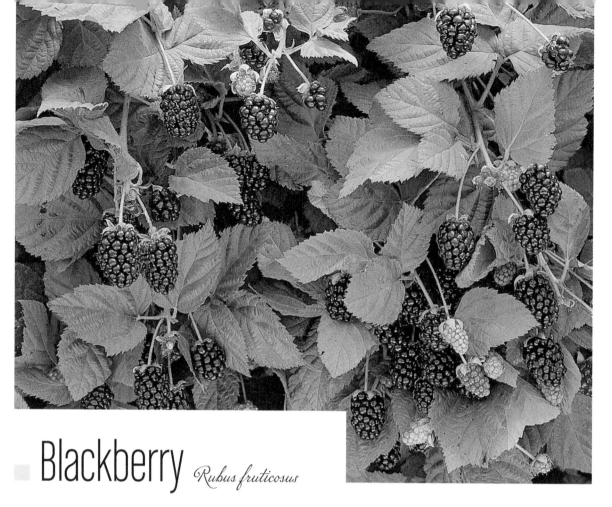

Blackberry *Rubus fruticosus*

There are few sights as satisfying in a medicinal garden or patch of wild-growing thicket as a wall of just-ripened berries. When we started our farm and had to rent greenhouse space, I was bringing decayed plant material out to the compost pile (one of those glamorous farm tasks) and came upon a 10-foot stretch of blackberries growing wild and unnoticed along an abandoned building. It was like finding out that Santa Claus is real. When you grow these plants, it's less of a happy surprise, but I think the feeling is always the same—pure, childlike delight, followed by fingers stained with berry juice. Blackberries, with their dark and shiny exteriors, are particularly gorgeous, and, although it's mainly the roots and leaves that are used in medicinal preparations, I'm guessing you can find a use for those berries too.

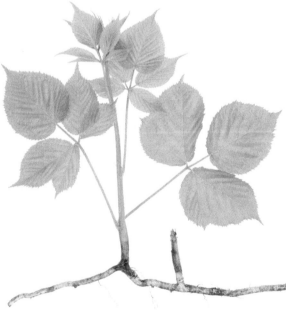

Blackberry stem, roots, and leaves—all can be used for medicinal purposes.

Because so much of the plant is used, blackberry can be used for an array of issues, from sore throats to minor burns. Some people have reported that blackberry can be used for more serious conditions as well, such as prostate problems, kidney issues, and anemia—but as always, have a chat with your physician about treating these conditions with herbs.

Here are a few ideas for your Rx/medicinal preparations:

- Create blackberry vinegar by covering a quart of berries with red wine vinegar and steep for a week in a cool, dark spot. Place a small plate inside the jar or bowl to keep berries submerged, which will prevent mold from forming. Strain and store the vinegar in the refrigerator, and use for treating coughs and sore throats.

- Eat the berries. Small sacrifice to pay for your health, right? Not only do the berries taste great, particularly in a smoothie, but they're also nutrition-packed and can be diuretic and internally cleansing. (Hint: that means don't eat too many, unless you need a *major* cleanse.)

- Dry the leaves, crush them with a mortar and pestle or coffee grinder, and brew them into a tea that can be used for indigestion or menstrual cramps.

CHECKLIST

Sun: Eight to ten hours per day

Shade: Full sun

Soil: Well-drained, loosened soil

Fertilizer: Use if plant seems to be struggling

Pests: Tend to be minimal, but look out for viruses

Water: Regularly, depending on soil dryness

Grow Indoors? No

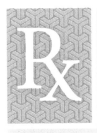

MEDICINE CABINET

Blackberry is not only delicious, but also a must-eat for its health properties. Plus, you use the leaves and roots as well, giving it extra points as a whole-plant remedy.

High in antioxidants

The wellness word du jour is "antioxidant," but it's not just a trend—an antioxidant is a molecule that inhibits oxidation, a process that can cause inflammation and other challenges in the body. In a study conducted by the U.S. Department of Agriculture, blackberries and certain black raspberries were found to have the highest antioxidant capacity of several berries tested.[1]

An array of medicinal uses

Not only are blackberries widespread geographically, but also boast a staggering array of medicinal benefits, according to researchers at the Institute of Pharmacy in India. The study notes that plants in the blackberry family are useful in the treatment of cancer, dysentery, diarrhea, whooping cough, colitis, toothache, anemia, psoriasis, sore throat, mouth ulcer, hemorrhoids, and minor bleeding.[2]

1. Wang, S.Y., Lin, H.S. "Antioxidant activity in fruits and leaves of blackberry, raspberry, and strawberry varies with cultivar and developmental stage." *Journal of Agricultural Food Chemistry*, 2000 Feb; 48(2): 140-6. http://www.ncbi.nlm.nih.gov/pubmed/10691606

2. Rameshwar, V., et al. "Rubus fruticosus (blackberry) use as an herbal medicine," *Pharmacognosy Review* 2014; 8(16): 01-104. http://www.ncbi.nlm.nih.gov/pmc/articles/PMC3992233/

PLANT·GROW·HARVEST·USE

When buying blackberry plants, you'll usually have the option of "summer bearing" or "fall bearing," which means exactly what it sounds like: berries in the summer or fall. You can also choose varieties that are thornless or thorny—although it makes sense that, as a home gardener, you'd want to avoid thorns as much as possible, the varieties that sport thorns can also be a deterrent for squirrels and other pests. Here are some options to consider:

- **Triple Crown:** With large berries, this thornless variety ripens early and has a good degree of winter hardiness. It tends to do best in warmer climates.
- **Ouachita:** A good option if you're looking to trellis the plants, and also comes as a thornless variety for warmer zones.
- **Natchez:** A newer variety developed by the University of Arkansas breeding program, this is the earliest ripening thornless variety, and has oblong berries.
- **Prime Jim:** A good option for cooler climates, this is a primocane variety, which means it will produce fruit in its first year of growth, although it's likely to be more abundant in the second onward.

PLANT For blackberries, which should produce fruit the second year from planting onward, site selection is crucial.

Choose a spot with full sun, since the bushes will thrive most with nice long days of sunshine. Most important, don't plant a new blackberry bush where any bramble-type plant has been before, such as other bushes or roses. Blackberries can be very vulnerable to disease that occurs as a result of a virus, and this can happen if problems have been building up in the soil over time. Also, wild blackberries can harbor viruses, so if you have both in your garden, keep them well separated from each other.

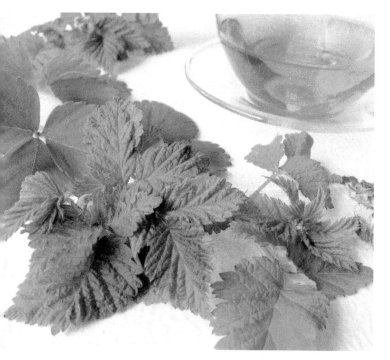

Blackberry leaves dry well for making into a tea.

Also, choose a spot that hasn't had members of the nightshade family (eggplants, peppers, tomatoes, and potatoes) growing there within the past couple years, since the remnants of those plants could potentially transmit a disease called verticillium wilt to the blackberries, with an emphasis on the "wilt."

Obtain blackberry plants from a nursery or reputable transplant grower, and when bringing them home, keep the plants cozy and wrapped until you're ready to plant (which, ideally, would be soon after buying them). Plant about 3 to 5 feet apart, and if doing multiple rows, plan on 6 to 10 feet between rows to permit bushy growth.

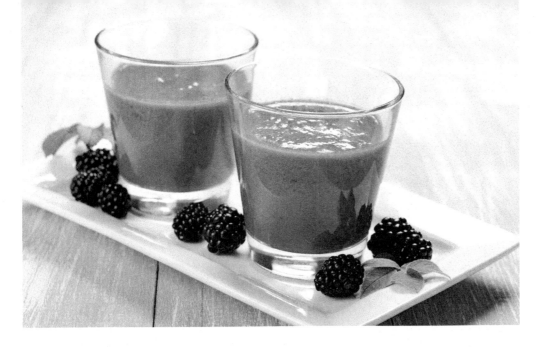

Fresh blackberries are delicious made into smoothies.

NUTRITIONAL VALUE OF BLACKBERRIES

per 100 g (3.5 oz)

Blackberries are rich in vitamin A, vitamin C, vitamin K, and potassium.

Energy	43 kcal
Carbohydrates	9.61 g
Dietary fiber	5.3 g
Fat	0.49 g
Protein	1.39 g
Water	88.15 g
Vitamin A	214 µg
Thiamine	0.02 mg
Riboflavin	0.026 mg
Niacin	0.646 mg
Vitamin B$_6$	0.03 mg
Folate	25 µg
Choline	0 mg
Vitamin C	21 mg
Vitamin E	1.17 mg
Vitamin K	19.8 µg
Calcium	29 mg
Iron	0.62 mg
Magnesium	20 mg
Cholesterol	0 mg
Phosphorus	22 mg
Potassium	162 mg
Sodium	1 mg
Zinc	0.53 mg

Source: USDA Nutrient Database

GROW Make sure to water well when you're first getting the plants established, and if you have the room, consider drip irrigation—this looks like a flat hose with small holes in it, which can be hooked up to a hose or spigot. The irrigation line delivers a regular amount of water to the plant without soaking the soil. You can improve soil moisture levels by mulching around the plants with leaves or chopped hay, and add some compost for a nice boost of fertilization.

Unless you're some kind of fruit whisperer (or get a variety classified as "primocane"), the plant won't bear fruit in the first year, but should provide blackberries in the second and subsequent years. Be sure to water well during the fruit development period, which you'll recognize by hard, white little berries appearing in early to midsummer. If the bushes seem to be getting out of control at any point, consider trellising them for easier harvest.

HARVEST & STORE Once you see those almost-berries, and slightly beforehand, pick some leaves for drying in order to make tea or decoctions. Once the berries form, all of the plant's energy goes toward that effort, making the leaves less potent in terms of medicinal properties.

To harvest the berries, just pick them like a delighted little kid who's seeing berries for the first time. Once they start fruiting, you'll be able to pick every three or four days, and harvesting this frequently will help to prevent birds from feasting more than you'd like.

With a well-established plant that's healthy and growing, you can afford to harvest some root bark as well. This has been noted as a good remedy for diarrhea, since the roots have an astringent effect on the digestive system, similar to witchhazel. Just boil the root bark in water for about twenty minutes, strain, and drink every couple hours until there's some relief. If the taste is too "rootbarky," add some honey.

Some people aren't fond of eating the hard center that can come with blackberries, but those get ground up beautifully in smoothies. You can also make jams, jellies, pies, or other desserts, although I'm always a bit dubious that a sugar-packed option will still hold medicinal properties. Worth a try, though, right?

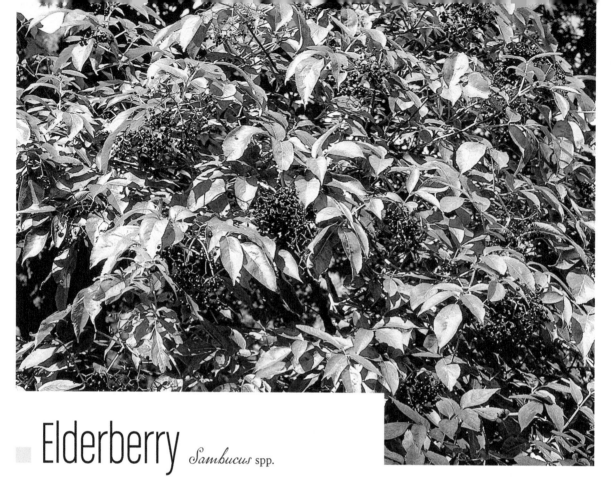

Elderberry *Sambucus* spp.

Sometimes found growing wild along roadsides and in abandoned fields, the elder plant has been called the "medicine chest of the country people" and almost every part can be used medicinally. Elder was often found in herb gardens in antiquity, and the Greeks and Romans used wood from the shrub to make musical instruments. It was once believed that if you stood under an elder plant at midnight during a midsummer night, you'd see the King of the Elves traveling nearby. Planting one near your house guarded you not only from thunder, but also witchcraft. (But not, apparently, from elf kings.) Beyond its mystical and medicinal uses, the berries have been used for jam, jelly, wine, pie, and elderberry cordial.

An infusion of elder flowers can be taken to treat respiratory issues, as well as flu and cold symptoms, while the berries can be made into a syrup that acts as a laxative. Even the bark can be employed for a diuretic.

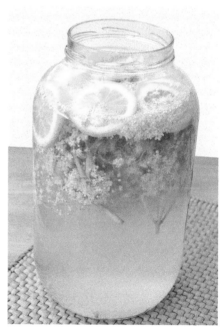

For a refreshing summer drink, try making an elderberry cordial.

Here are a few ideas for your Rx/medicinal preparations:

- To address digestive issues, particularly constipation, make a decoction of the elderberry bark by harvesting a young branch, stripping the bark from it, and simmering for about an hour. Strain, and start with a small amount of a few tablespoons. When it comes to herbs with laxative properties, you'll want to keep amounts modest at first until you know how it works for your body.
- For colds, use dried or fresh blossoms in an infusion, and combine with peppermint or yarrow for an additional immunity boost.
- To create a general tonic, boil fresh berries in water for two to three minutes, and then strain the resulting juice through cheesecloth or a fine-meshed sieve. Combine with a touch of honey to remove its sourness and store in a glass jar in the fridge. Drink a small glass of the syrup diluted with water (to taste) and again, only drink a small amount until you know how it affects your system.

PLANT·GROW·HARVEST·USE

Sporting creamy white flowers in early summer, the elderberry shrub spends all season leisurely turning its berries into a deep purple, almost black, by autumn. Considered one of the easiest and

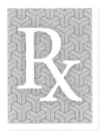

MEDICINE CABINET

Elderberry shrubs boast a wealth of black berries that ripen in late summer and boast a significant amount of antioxidants and vitamins. The fruit and its leaves have been prized for flu relief in addition to supporting general wellness.

Effective for the flu

Researchers noted the elderberry has been used in folk medicine for centuries to treat influenza, colds, and sinusitis, and it has been reported to have antiviral activity against influenza and herpes simplex. In investigating the efficacy of elderberry syrup, they found that patients suffering from influenza-type symptoms found relief about four days earlier than those on a placebo syrup. They noted that the extract seems to offer an efficient, safe, and cost-effective treatment for influenza.[1]

Plenty of antioxidants

Elderberries are rich in health-promoting phytochemicals such as polyphenols and anthocyanins, and display a significant antioxidant activity, noted researchers.[2]

1. Zakay-Rones, Z., et al. "Randomized study of the efficacy and safety of oral elderberry extract in the treatment of influenza A and B virus infections," *J Int Med Res* 2004 Mar-Apr; 32(2)132-40. http://www.ncbi.nlm.nih.gov/pubmed/15080016

2. Jimenez, P., et al. "Effects of short-term heating on total polyphenols, anthocyanins, antioxidant activity and lectins of different parts of dwarf elder (Sambucus ebulus L.)," *Plant Foods Hum Nutr.*, 2014 Jun; 69(2):168-74. http://www.ncbi.nlm.nih.gov/pubmed/24793353

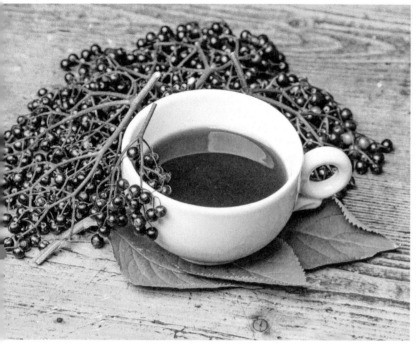

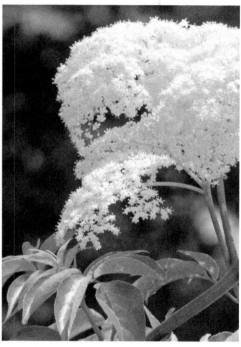

Left: Elderberry tea is often used as a general wellness tonic.

Right: Elderberry's flowers make a nice ornamental touch to any garden.

most versatile shrubs to grow, these antioxidant-packed plants have been used for making fermented beverages like cordials and wines, in addition to all types of preserves. Depending on variety, the leaves can vary between green and purple, with pink flowers that create a nice border if used for ornamental purposes.

VARIETIES When it comes to elder varieties, there are three main types: European elderberry (*Sambucus nigra*) grows up to 20 feet tall, blooms early and does well in cooler climates, down to Zone 4; American elderberry (*S. canadensis*) is a wild species often found growing in meadows, along prairies, and occasionally, in abandoned spaces; red elderberry (*S. racemosa*) has poisonous berries that should not be eaten, even cooked. Although I believe you shouldn't plant *S. racemosa* at all, it's important to include it in this list so you know what to avoid if you're shopping at the local greenhouse or nursery and come across this option. With that in mind, here are a few choices:

- **Adams:** Large, dark purple fruits that ripen in August and are particularly good for pies, jams, and jellies. Although this American variety is sometimes designated as Adams No. 1 and Adams No. 2, there isn't a significant difference between the two.
- **Black Beauty:** A European variety that features striking purple foliage and lemon-scented flowers.
- **York:** An American variety that produces the largest elderberry of all the available varieties. Since it grows only about 6 feet tall, it can be better for more modest garden plans.

PLANT Like other types of berry plants, elderberries fruit best when they're at least a few years old. Also, they fruit beautifully if you plant at least two different varieties within 60 feet of each other.

When planning your garden, keep size in mind: these plants can easily get 10 to 20 feet tall and are full shrubs. They can make ideal ornamentals—as long as you can keep them trimmed back properly.

Choose a spot that's either full sun or partial shade, with slightly acidic soil, although that's less important than finding soil that stays consistently moist. To help keep roots well irrigated, consider using a layer of compost around roots, followed by a layer of mulch. Space plants 6 to 10 feet apart, depending on how large the variety is expected at maturity.

If your soil has a heavy clay component, consider planting the shrubs in a raised bed, where they grow very well, especially when pruned properly to maintain shape.

Plant in spring, and if you can't find an elderberry cutting or roots locally (ask around first, isn't that why social media was created?), there are several elderberry nursery providers online. Just be sure to contact the nurseries in the *early* part of the year so you can time delivery to coincide with your planting schedule.

GROW Elderberries can thrive for years, but should be fertilized annually to grow best. Put a thin layer of compost around the roots followed by mulch like woodchips, straw, or hay.

Every year, a plant will send out new branches that will fruit heavily the season after, ensuring that you'll have a steady supply of fruit. Once you notice branches that have been in place for over three years, and are declining in productivity, prune those and remove to make space for newer growth.

Also, stay on top of weeding, since weeds can be a problem for elderberry plants if they get too numerous.

HARVEST & STORE Different parts of the elder plant are harvested during certain times: the flowers before they open, the leaves in midsummer, elderberries when they ripen to a dark purple color in late summer, and roots in the fall before the first frost.

When harvesting fruit, clip off the entire cluster into a bowl and put into the refrigerator, since the berries don't store well at room temperature.

One *very important note* when it comes to elderberries: ripe, cooked berries of most varieties are edible, but only one variety, *Sambucus nigra,* has berries that are non-toxic in raw form. A good rule of thumb is always to cook the berries for culinary or medicinal use.

In terms of using the parts of the plant, fresh flowers can be used for an infusion, while dried flowers and leaves make an excellent tea, especially when combined with a sweeter herb like mint. When using bark or roots, dry them on a screen until they're crisp enough to snap. Then, you can create a decoction that can be stored in the fridge and use as a tonic, particularly for digestive issues. You can also make a poultice out of fresh leaves by creating a mash and applying directly to bruises, sprains, and wounds.

As with other herbs, store any leftover components in airtight glass jars and put in a cool, dark place.

NUTRITIONAL VALUE OF ELDERBERRIES
The nutritional value of elderberries has not been established.

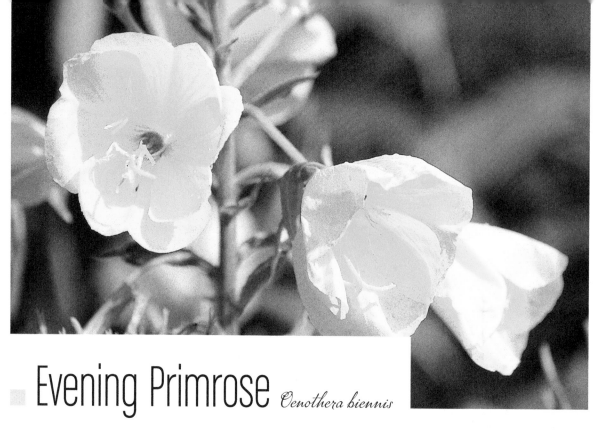

Evening Primrose *Oenothera biennis*

One of the few biennial herbs, evening primrose has been garnering attention recently for its promising medicinal value, with research in the 1980s first noting that this herb can alleviate effects of menopause and pre-menstrual syndrome. After that revelation, herbalists began taking a closer look at its properties and found that evening primrose contains useful fatty acids, including gamma-linolenic acid, which can balance female hormones. Newer research has begun to expand the herb's promise, and it's now considered a good candidate for issues related to bowel health, depression, hyperactivity, and other issues. Plus, the herb features bright yellow flowers that open at twilight—giving it the "evening" part of its name—making it a garden showoff just as other plants and flowers are closing up for the night.

Evening primrose is very potent as an essential oil, and in that form, it's been used to relieve chronic stress and lower blood pressure. But the herb can be utilized in other forms for a range of uses.

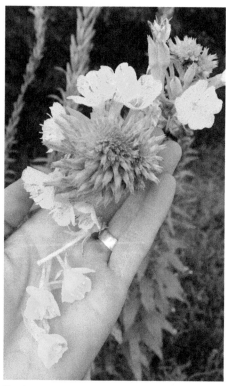

Evening primrose blooms at twilight, but is still in flower in the morning.

Here are a few ideas for your Rx/medicinal preparations:

- To soothe a nagging dry cough, make an infusion by combining a teaspoon of dried evening primrose leaves and the peeled outer skin of the stems together with just-boiled water and let steep for 15 minutes. Strain and drink a small glass, then another a few hours later.
- For a general anti-anxiety tonic, create a decoction by combining an ounce of dried evening primrose root and simmering for about an hour. Strain, cool, and drink a cup before a meal.
- To alleviate pain from arthritis or other inflammatory issues, dry the leaves and flowers and make a tea; drink three times per day for a few days, until you find relief.

PLANT·GROW·HARVEST·USE

Opening in the early evening to attract moths, evening primrose flowers might be small, but their colors really pop in the twilight. Another advantage: the biennial plant grows quickly, lasts for years, and self-seeds rapidly. The plant actually grows as a wildflower in many parts of the US—it's one of the few native wildflowers in North America—and is sometimes considered a weed, but likely, that's only by people who haven't sat gazing at its flowers opening as the sunset begins.

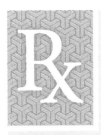
Evening primrose is often used to relieve itchiness on irritated skin, even for chronic conditions like dermatitis and eczema. Some herbalists have also recommended the herb for symptoms related to premenstrual syndrome and rheumatoid arthritis.

Helpful for gastric system

Evening primrose oil was administered to rats fed a standard chow diet as well as gastric system inhibitors, such as non-steroidal, anti-inflammatory drugs. The results showed the herb's oil provided significant protection against gastric damage.[1]

Beneficial for rheumatologic conditions

For those with rheumatoid arthritis, diets rich in pro-inflammatory foods, combined with use of non-steroidal, anti-inflammatory drugs (such as Motrin or Aleve) can aggravate symptoms. Researchers found that evening primrose oil and borage oil both show some promise in reducing inflammation and that results suggest some clinical benefits to the treatments.[2]

1. al-Sabanah, O.A. "Effect of evening primrose oil on gastric ulceration and secretion induced by various ulcerogenic and necrotizing agents in rats," *Food Chem Toxicol.* 1997; 35(8):769-775 http://www.ncbi.nlm.nih.gov/pubmed/9350221
2. Belch, J.J., et al. "Evening primrose oil and borage oil in rheumatologic conditions," *Am. J. Clin. Nutr.* 2000;71(1Suppl): 352S-356S. http://www.ncbi.nlm.nih.gov/pubmed/10617996

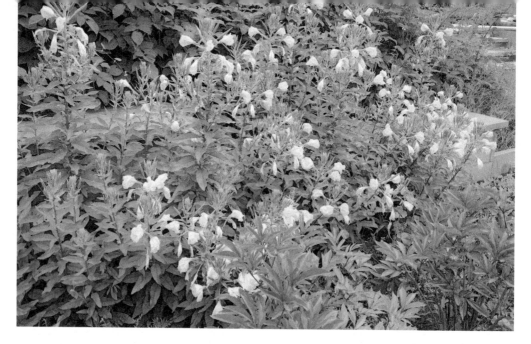

Not only is evening primrose medicinal, but it's a nice ornamental as well.

VARIETIES When selecting an evening primrose variety, the choice usually depends on the plant's flowers, which can range from a cheery white to a sultry orange. In general, though, it may be hard to choose—evening primrose flowers are gorgeous, and the fact that they bloom just as sunset is brimming over the horizon makes them even more magical. Best of all, they all have medicinal properties as well as ornamental appeal.

- **Missouri**: One of the classic evening primrose varieties, with bright yellow flowers that bloom from June to September. Considered winter hardy to Zone 4 and boasts velvet-textured leaves that make the plant gorgeous in ornamental landscapes.
- **Glowing Magenta**: Slightly smaller than Missouri, and with deep rose-colored flowers, this variety tends to be favored for container gardening. Better for warmer climates since it's winter hardy only to Zone 5.
- **Sunset Boulevard**: Just like the classic movie, but without being crushingly depressing or involving mentally unstable former celebrities. The variety has beautiful, cup-shaped blooms the start as yellow (think of an ingénue) then mature into deep, complicated shades of red and apricot.
- **Innocence**: Lovely white flowers with a splash of central yellow make this variety a stunner in any garden. Good for borders, and especially nice in large containers.

PLANT Because evening primrose establishes so easily, it can become invasive if not kept under control, so when planning where the plant will fit in your garden space, choose enough room where you can maintain it through pruning. Raised beds work well, since they contain the sprawl if you happen to get behind on garden maintenance.

Choose a spot in full sun (although the plant can tolerate partial shade if necessary) and make sure soil drains well. This herb isn't particularly fussy about the richness of the soil, but its roots suffer if they're encased in a more clay-like environment.

Unlike some plants that do well being propagated through division, evening primrose doesn't always succeed when transplanted, so plant from seed instead, especially since that tactic is ridiculously simple.

Sow the seeds in late spring, and cover lightly. It's easiest to simply spread them like wildflowers instead of planting in rows. If you live in a warmer area, you can plant in autumn as well. Germination time will vary depending on conditions, but usually takes between one week and one month. When the plants start to come up, thin them out so you don't have an area that's too bushy.

GROW Evening primrose is one of those plants that does well with benign neglect, some of my favorite kind. Water during periods of drought, but otherwise be cautious not to overwater, since this will negatively affect the roots.

Because the plant self-seeds so rapidly, limit growth by snapping off the flowers regularly—which you'd do anyway to use them for medicinal preparations—and thin the plants if needed.

Some gardeners achieve control through trellising, which can also achieve a nice ornamental effect alongside a house or beside a patio.

HARVEST & STORE All parts of the evening primrose plant can be used, and some people prepare the roots like potatoes, by boiling them gently until they soften and slicing them up. Serve with your favorite condiment, perhaps?

The plant follows the harvest schedule of other herbs in terms of medicinal potency: harvest leaves and stems first, before the flowers begin to appear, and dry on a clean mesh screen for teas and tinctures; harvest flowers after they've been blooming for a few weeks, and dry those as well; and harvest roots in the fall when the plant has begun to die back and starts putting all its energy into the roots for hibernation.

You can also eat the stems raw in salads, especially the young shoots that you've thinned as a way to control the plant's spread.

The parts of the plant used commercially are the seeds, which are harvested from the flowers and then made into evening primrose oil. This oil is the most studied part of the plant, and has been touted as the most sensational preventive discovery since vitamin C, since it contains pain-relieving compounds that can ease a range of maladies. Although the creation of essential oil isn't covered in this book since I wouldn't trust my skills with a home distillation setup (in other words, I'd probably blow up the house), if you're the chemistry-loving type who can expertly work a distillation process, then evening primrose seeds would be a great choice for essential oil creation.

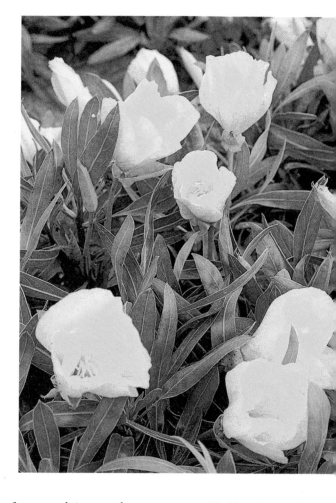

The Missouri variety of evening primrose, with velvet-textured leaves.

NUTRITIONAL VALUE OF EVENING PRIMROSE

The nutritional value of evening primrose has not been established.

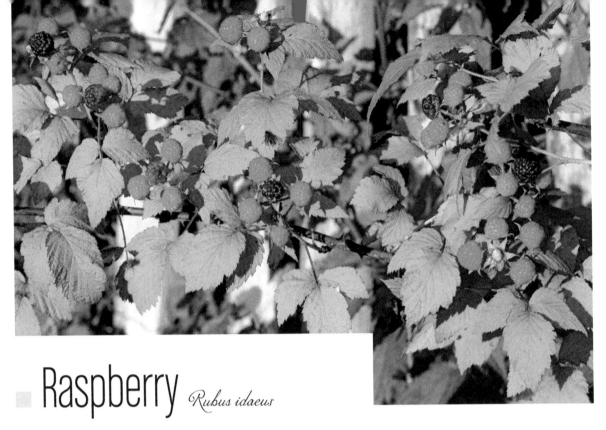

Raspberry *Rubus idaeus*

During the long, long winters in Minnesota, sometimes I dream of raspberries. Literally. Although blueberries and blackberries hold their places in my heart, there's something about the squishy, delicate raspberries that let me know midsummer has truly arrived, and it's glorious! An added benefit to all that dreamy fruit is the incredible leaves, which have been used for generations by European and Native American women to address issues related to menstrual cycles, pregnancy, and general uterine health. Sometimes called the "woman's herb," raspberry is a relative of the rose, and both the leaves and fruit are rich in vitamins and minerals, as well as antioxidants. It's also one of the few herbs that's recommended during pregnancy, to help ensure a smoother labor process.

Of all the herbs I drink in tea form, raspberry leaf tastes the most like a traditional black tea to me. Sometimes I even add milk and sugar since I forget it's an herbal. The leaves are high in magnesium, potassium, and iron, making them helpful for everything from leg cramps to nausea.

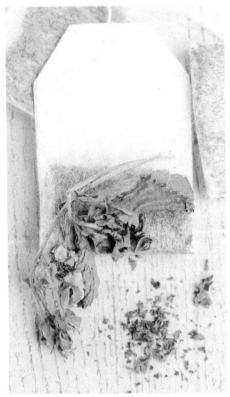

Dried raspberry leaves work well as a simple tea.

Here are a few ideas for your Rx/medicinal preparations:

◆ As a general tonic, pick some leaves during the early part of the season and dry on a clean mesh screen; crumble or grind and place into tea bags.

◆ Create an infusion by pouring just-boiled water over dried or fresh leaves, and allow to steep for 15 minutes. Soak a clean cloth in the liquid and then place that over sunburn or rashes.

◆ For symptoms of gum disease, make a tincture by steeping dried raspberry leaf in alcohol for two weeks; strain, and use as a mouthwash.

PLANT·GROW·HARVEST·USE

Raspberries are one of those plants that makes me swoony. Unlike blackberries, with their hard little core, raspberries are so tender and sweet. Like many berries, they're incredibly versatile when it comes to cooking and baking (or dropping into glasses of champagne), and they have the added lure of a short growing season, so eating them feels like a rare treat. Plus, you get leaves that are uniquely geared for medicinal preparations. All this, and easy to grow? That's a charmer.

VARIETIES Although raspberries are suited for cooler climates, plant hybrid experts have developed several varieties that can be grown in warmer zones as well. Most people are familiar with the type

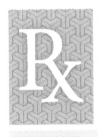

MEDICINE CABINET

Although raspberry's fruits are tantalizing and nutritious, the part of the plant most used for medicinal effect is the leaf, which is often made into tea for gastrointestinal disorders, and respiratory system issues.

Helpful for contractions during labor

Researchers noted that studies on raspberry leaf extract from the 1940s had shown a beneficial effect on their labor and contractions, but the precise nature of the effect wasn't specified. In examining the constituent properties of the herb, they found that the extract is "able to modify the course of labor favorably by producing more coordinated uterine contractions."[1]

Anti-obesity effect

Raspberry ketone is a chemical derived from red raspberries, and has been used for weight loss and obesity treatment, as well as an aid to increase lean body mass. One study found that raspberry ketones prevent and improve obesity and fatty liver.[2]

1. Bamford, D.S, et al. "Raspberry leaf tea: a new aspect to an old problem," *Br J Pharmacol* 1970; 40:161P-162P. http://www.ncbi.nlm.nih.gov/pmc/articles/PMC1702706/

2. Morimoto, C. "Anti-obese action of raspberry ketone," *Life Sci* 2005; 77:194-204.

that produces bright red berries, but there are other choices as well, and it can be fun to grow different varieties tucked in close to each other. Quick note when choosing: there are two types of raspberries. The summer-bearing kind is true to its name, bearing one crop in midsummer, while the ever-bearing has two growing periods, one in summer and then another in fall.

- **Prelude:** A summer-bearing plant that ripens in mid-June in certain zones, making it the earliest berry of the season. This is a good choice for putting near plants that ripen in midsummer, so you can have a long berry season.
- **Bristol:** A summer-bearing black raspberry variety that grows upright and has tight cluster formation, making it easy to harvest.
- **Mac Black:** Another summer-bearing variety, but this one ripens in late season, with black raspberries. A good candidate for trellising.
- **Anne:** More of an ever-bearer, but with the majority of fruit appearing in the fall. This variety is unusual since the berries are a pale yellow color.

When harvesting, look for raspberry leaves that are free of blemishes or pest damage.

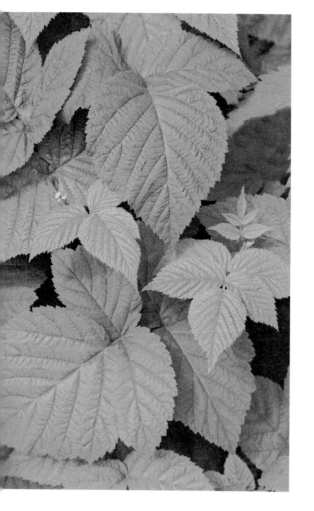

PLANT When choosing a spot for raspberry plants, find one with full sun and slightly acidic to neutral soil, which means the pH should be about 7 or lower. If it's much higher, add in some amendments that will "sour up" the soil, such as coffee grounds or granular sulfur. Work these into the soil, along with some compost, at least a few weeks prior to planting if possible. If you're the kind of person who's great with planning, work into the soil the autumn before you plant.

Many nurseries sell young raspberry plants, and there are some great and reputable nurseries online, especially those that specialize in berry plants. Just be sure to place your order early in the year because they have a tendency to sell out.

Because raspberries do better with a high amount of moisture, soak the roots (not the leaves) in water for a few hours before planting. This will help get moisture into the plant more effectively, and ensure a better transplanting process.

Dig a hole that allows the roots enough room to spread, and place raspberry root in there, with leaves just above ground. Space plants about 3 feet apart, and if you're doing multiple rows, space those at least 8 feet apart since the bushes will get full and putting them too close will make harvesting into a chore.

Many people create a trellis or staking system to support the plant, or plant along a fence line where you can tie the plants to the fence. This works well with chain link fences in particular.

GROW Once raspberry plants have established and are growing nicely, there's minimal maintenance beyond making sure they're

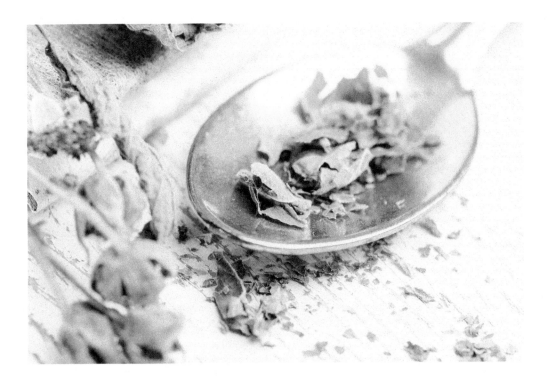

Raspberry leaves dry easily and can be crumpled by hand for teas.

NUTRITIONAL VALUE OF RASPBERRIES

per 100 g (3.5 oz)

Raspberries are rich in folate, choline, vitamin E, vitamin K, calcium, iron, magnesium, zinc, and potassium.

Energy	52 kcal
Carbohydrates	11.94 g
Dietary fiber	6.5 g
Fat	0.65 g
Protein	1.20 g
Water	85.75 g
Vitamin A	2 µg
Thiamine	0.032 µg
Riboflavin	0.038 mg
Niacin	0.598 mg
Vitamin B$_6$	0.550 µg
Folate	21 µg
Choline	0 mg
Vitamin C	26.2 mg
Vitamin E	0.87 mg
Vitamin K	7.8 µg
Calcium	25 mg
Iron	0.69 mg
Magnesium	22 mg
Manganese	0 mg
Phosphorus	29 mg
Potassium	151 mg
Sodium	1 mg
Zinc	0.42 mg

Source: USDA Nutrient Database

well-watered. Many growers have found the plants do well with mulching throughout the season, which helps keep the roots healthy and prevents disease issues. Also be sure to weed regularly, since berry plants do better when they don't have to compete with weeds.

HARVEST & STORE To use raspberry leaf, simply pick the leaves at any point during the season. Be sure to look closely at the leaves to make sure they're free of any spots, insect eggs, or signs of powdery mildew (which looks like talcum powder), so that you're collecting only the healthiest leaves.

Like other leaves, dry on a clean mesh screen. Since raspberry plants have larger leaves, I sometimes use a cooling rack, similar to one you'd utilize for cookies or breads, since this can speed up the drying process. When the leaves are completely dry, use a spice grinder or crumble with your hands, and store in an airtight glass jar in a dark cupboard.

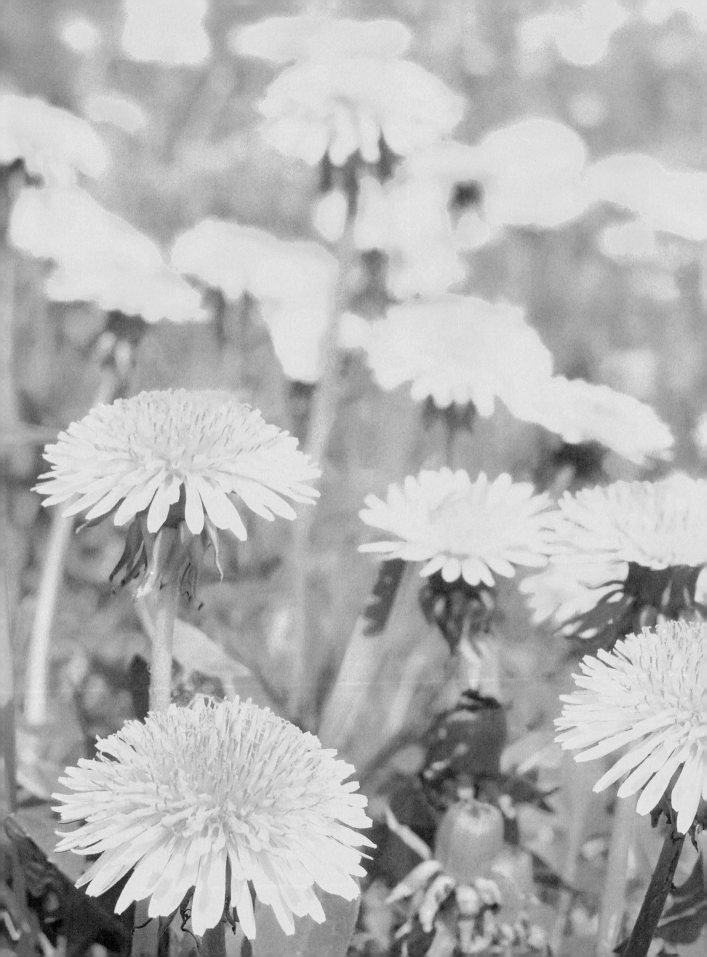

SIX

Wild Yard Friends

Although the previous chapters covered just a fraction of potentially useful plants—perhaps setting you on a path to expand your garden even more—I'd also like to make a plea to consider the non-cultivated options that might be growing in and around your carefully planted beds.

What many people consider weeds could be the start of a beautiful herbal relationship. Once you start recognizing these once-reviled weeds, you'll begin to see your yard in a whole new way. For me, it took just an hour-long class on local herbs for me to get hooked on finding wild medicinal plants. The speaker mentioned that plantain (which is covered here later, but trust me, it's very cool) could be used for insect bites and wounds, and that it was so abundant in the city that we'd all probably see some on our walk back to the parking lot. Sure, I thought, dubiously.

I saw plantain about five steps out the door, and now I see it wherever I go. It was like learning there's a new color.

Now, I walk through the meadows around our farm and spot an array of medicinal options, knowing that there are probably dozens more that I've failed to identify (yet!). But you don't need to have large field spaces to take advantage of wild choices—I've seen just as many useful "weeds" when I walk around my former neighborhood in South Minneapolis.

Here are ten wild plants that are often saved from my lawnmower's wrath, with many making their way into our medicine chest.

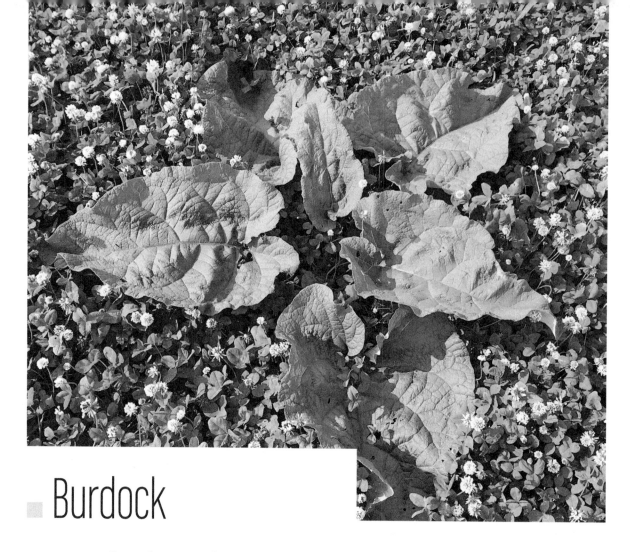

Burdock

Known for its anti-inflammatory and antibacterial properties, burdock also contains some powerful antioxidants. The plant is a diuretic and the roots can act as a laxative. Some people make nettle, dandelion, and burdock beer as a midsummer tonic.

- **Identify:** Once you spot burdock, you'll see it everywhere. The stout, common weed has enormous leaves and stems when mature, and can sport purple flowers that bloom between June and October. The heart-shaped leaves are green on top and whitish on the bottom, making identification easier. The stalks closely resemble rhubarb.

- **Harvest:** Leave the especially large burdock alone and concentrate instead on the smaller, younger plants that are less bitter. You'll be using the stalk, so discard the leaves.

- **Use:** Its roots can be eaten, but it's usually the stalks that are a better choice, once they're peeled and boiled for about twenty minutes. If you're a fan of bitter foods, try eating the leaves by steaming them and then serving with other wild greens.

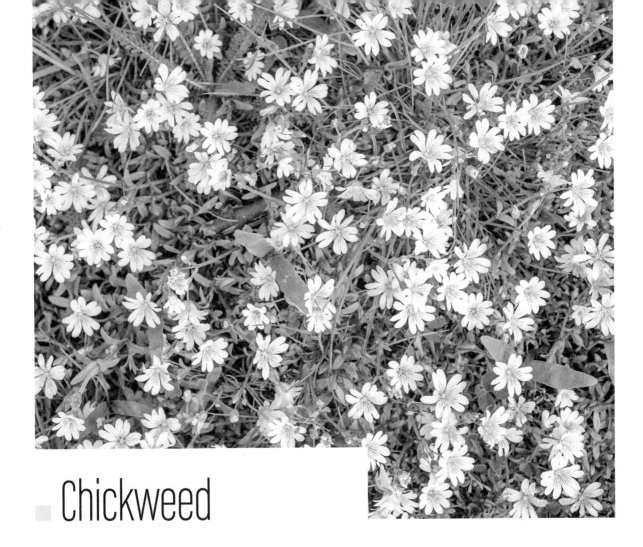

Chickweed

Chickweed gets it name because chickens gravitate toward it. Humans use this herb mainly for skin issues, with a poultice of chickweed seen as helpful for cuts and bruises, but herbalists have also used the plant for arthritis, menstrual pain, and bronchitis.

- **Identify:** Usually fairly small, chickweed is only a few inches tall and has tiny, oval leaves that grow in pairs. A fine line of hair extends on one side of a thin stem. When blooming, the plant has white, five-part flowers.
- **Harvest:** Clip the majority of the plant, being sure to leave the bottom of the plant so it can regrow.
- **Use:** For external preparations, chop up chickweed stems and leaves and grind them into a paste. Apply on affected areas, covered with a clean bandage. You can also make a tea by pouring boiling water over fresh leaves and steeping for fifteen minutes. Chickweed makes a nice spring green, and tastes like spinach when it's steamed.

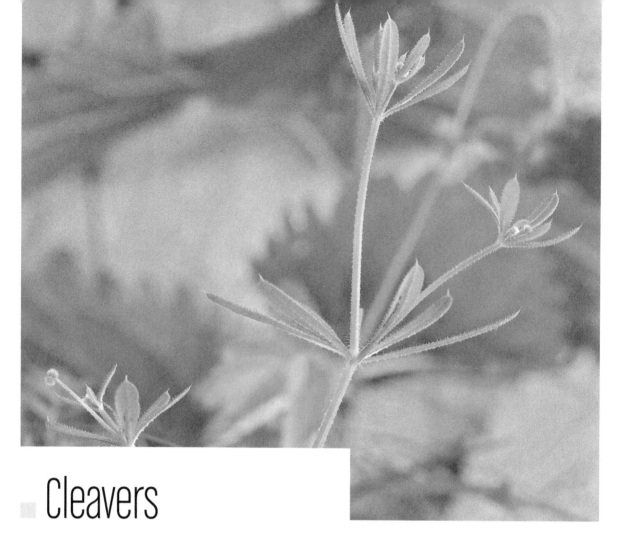

Cleavers

In terms of alternate names, cleavers might win the prize in any "also known as" competition, with other designations like goosegrass, barweed, grip grass, scratweed, and even the charming robin-run-in-the-grass. The herb has diuretic properties, and is also used to detoxify the digestive system and stimulate the lymphatic system.

- **Identify**: Cleavers are covered in small hooks that cling to whatever they touch. The leaves are small and thin, and appear in a whorled pattern around the stem.
- **Harvest**: Most likely, the cleavers will grab onto you, so all you have to do is gently remove them from your clothes and collect them. Put them into a clean muslin or plastic bag, as opposed to anything containing other herbs, or you'll have a sticky mess.
- **Use**: Cleavers are best when eaten as young plants in the spring, because they become woody and tough later in the season. Throw into salads or smoothies to eat raw, or steam for ten minutes with other spring greens.

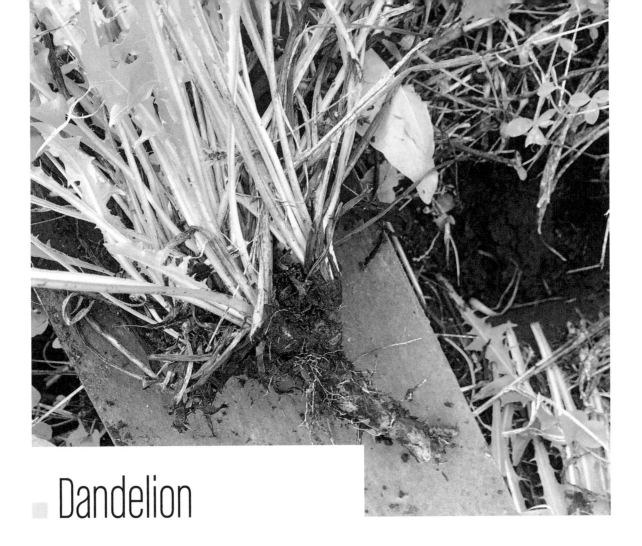

Dandelion

If there's one weed that seems to be the most combatted, and yet the most resilient, it's the humble dandelion. Although the scourge of lawn-loving homeowners everywhere, the dandelion is rich in beta-carotene, vitamin C, and numerous minerals. It boasts more protein than spinach, and has been used for thousands of years to treat anemia, depression, skin issues, and scurvy.

Identify: You're kidding, right? But just in case you've never seen one, dandelions have long, spiked leaves and cheerful, bright yellow flowers on a single stalk. When they bolt, the flowers turn into white globes of fluffy seeds that float toward whatever neighbor resents you the most.

Harvest: Every part of the plant is edible, so you can pick leaves, blooms, stems, and even roots. They tend to have a bitter flavor in midsummer, so minimize that taste by harvesting in spring or fall.

Use: Dandelion greens are delicious when lightly braised with butter, or included raw in a salads. The leaves can be dried and made into tea, and the flowers make a nice edible flower in a dish like risotto.

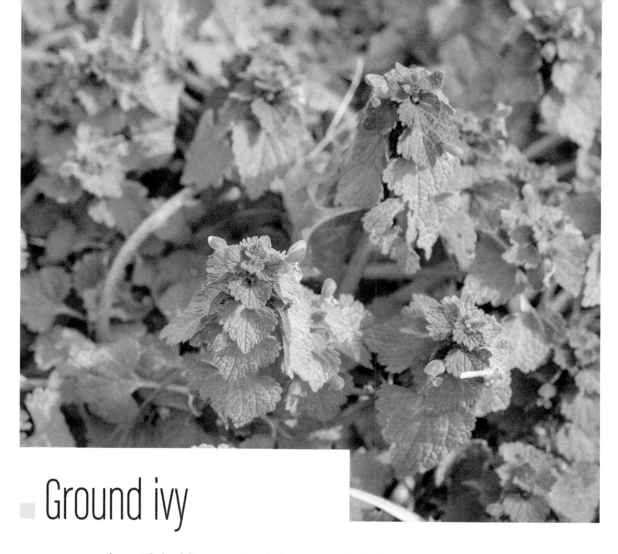

Ground ivy

Along with dandelion, ground ivy is the scourge of picky homeowners everywhere. Although the plant is small, it's remarkably invasive and can take over an entire lawn if left unchecked. Traditionally, ground ivy has been used to treat constipation, coughs, kidney issues, and sciatica. Some practitioners roll up fresh leaves and insert into the nose to alleviate headaches.

Identify: Unlike some forms of ivy—the type that crawl up houses and prestigious universities—ground ivy has scalloped leaves and small purple flowers. When crushed or mowed, the plant gives off a minty aroma.

Harvest: Pick off leaves, or cut some shoots so you get several leaves. Older ground ivy is usually bitter, so if you're looking to include it in an edible mix, choose smaller leaves. The older leaves still have plenty of medicinal clout, so if you want to use it for tea, select those leaves and dry them.

Use: Make tea once the herbs are dried, or add to soups or other cooked dishes. Cooking will take out most of the bitter taste. If you're a home brewer, try adding some to beer, which is said to increase a beer's shelf life.

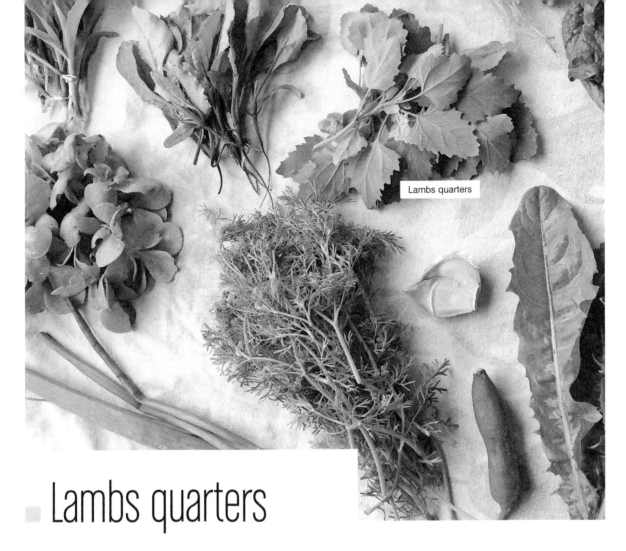

Lambs quarters

Lambs quarters

With their jagged leaves and slender stalks, lambs quarters tend to get passed by because they're so abundant, and have a "weedy" look to them. But this relative to spinach and beets is packed with vitamins and minerals and has been used to address digestion issues and stomach aches.

- **Identify**: With a slightly white coating on the leaves, lambs quarters often looks dusty at first glance. When mature, the plant has tiny green flowers that cluster on top.
- **Harvest**: Pick off leaves, as you would with spinach or leaf lettuce. Its seeds and flowers are also edible. Make sure the area where you're harvesting is known to be uncontaminated; lambs quarters often appear on toxic soil, as nature's way of attempting to restore nutrients.
- **Use**: For most of the early summer, we throw lambs quarters into salads, or lightly sauté the leaves in coconut oil to put on top of tacos. The plant has an earthy taste, similar to collards, but with a slightly lemony undertone. Because lambs quarters are so good for digestion, it makes sense to eat them to get the most medicinal clout.

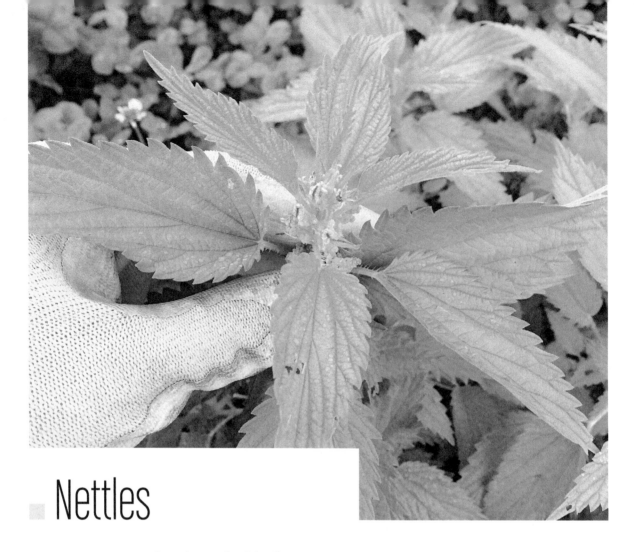

Nettles

Outstanding when used to fight allergies, nettles (sometimes called stinging nettles) are usually abundant in both urban and rural settings. Just when I was planning on going out to forage them in the woods, I realized I had some growing under my flowering cherry tree.

- **Identify**: Nettles can grow fairly tall—up to 7 feet—and have sawtooth-type leaves that look a bit like lemon balm when they're small. The plant flowers annually with small greenish or brownish blooms.
- **Harvest**: Take the leaves for drying, and keep the name in mind when harvesting. Once, I tried picking leaves without wearing gloves and the few stings I received made my hand throb for hours. Harvest in May or June, before the flowers appear.
- **Use**: Dry the leaves and make into a tea. I drink this every spring to combat pollen allergies, and it works like a charm. The tea also boasts antioxidants, and can be made with fresh nettles. If you're adding it to culinary dishes, steam the leaves briefly and include with other spring greens.

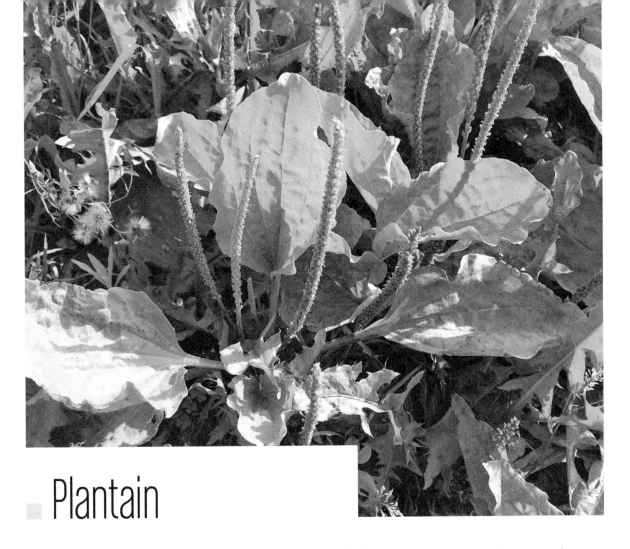

Plantain

Pronounced the same way as the large, banana-like fruit that's a staple in tropical countries, plantain is a humble herb with significant power for medicinal use. Applied to a wound, the chewed leaves can slow or stop bleeding, heal burns, and take the itch out of insect bites.

- **Identify**: With rounded leaves and a small central spire that looks like a little brush, plantain is easy to spot, especially because it tends to be abundant.
- **Harvest**: Because plantain is so common on lawns, in sidewalk cracks, and alongside walkways, it's important to make sure the area hasn't been chemically treated before harvesting. If you're sure that it's clean, pick the leaves.
- **Use**: As a topical application, plantain provides immediate relief for burning and itching caused by insect bites or allergic reactions to poison ivy. Simply pick a leaf, chew it to release the plant's anti-inflammatory properties, and apply the wet, lumpy result to any irritation.

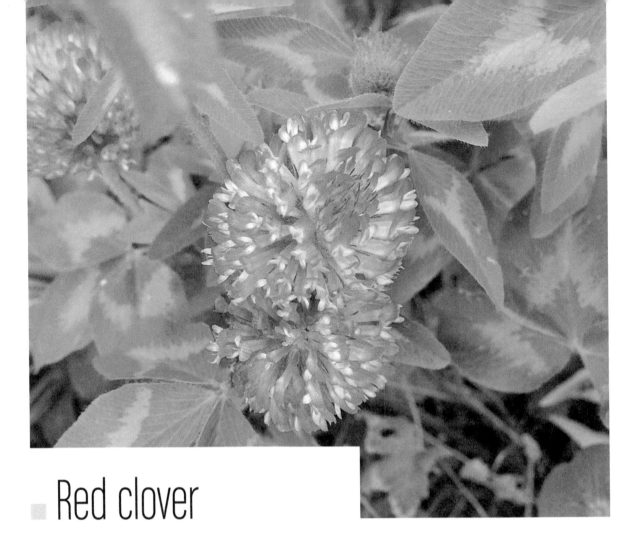

Red clover

Although red clover is sometimes classified as a weed, it's actually the national flower of Denmark, and has been used for a wide range of maladies, including coughs, cancer, respiratory issues, and lymphatic system disorders.

- **Identify**: Red clover has a distinctive, small flower that can vary from dark pink to light purple. The leaves are clustered in threes and have a pale crescent line in the middle.
- **Harvest**: For medicinal use, pick the flower tops and place on a clean cloth or in a paper bag poked with air holes for drying. Or preserve them fresh by placing them in an airtight container in a refrigerator.
- **Use**: Red clover's flowers are edible, and make a nice pop of color to summer salads, as well as giving the dish some medicinal power. I've also thrown one on top of lemonade for guests, and added them as garnish alongside cooked dishes. To make a tea, dry the flowers and crumble into a tea bag.

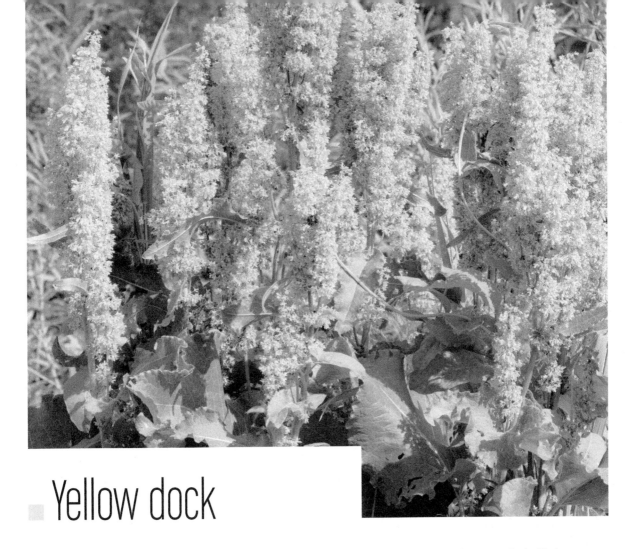

Yellow dock

Much like cleavers, yellow dock has an array of other names, including sheep sorrel, chukkah, narrow dock, curly dock, and romaza. The herb has been used for dermatitis, scurvy, and bacterial infections. Mainly, though, it's helpful for digestive issues and is stellar at treating constipation.

- **Identify**: The plant features a tall flower stalk with yellow, sometimes clustered, blooms. Leaves are long and pointed at the top, and also appear in clusters.
- **Harvest**: For medicinal use, dig up part of yellow dock's roots (which, true to its name, are yellow) while making sure to leave enough rootstock to keep the plant healthy. Also harvest the leaf stalks for fresh dishes. Harvest in late summer or autumn, after the plants have fully seeded, as an added measure of sustainable harvesting.
- **Use**: Yellow dock's leaf stalks make a nice addition to salads, or you can also grind them up and combine them with toothpaste as a way to address gingivitis. To use the roots, dry them in a well-ventilated area and then create a tincture that can be taken for a few days to treat constipation.

Miscellaneous Garden Supplies

Even when you're working to keep costs in line, it seems there's always just one more thing to buy at the garden center. Maybe you want to try some coconut coir to mix into your soil to improve drainage, or you're loving those glass watering bulbs that can be stuck into a pot and left for days. When I'm trying to stick to a budget, I try to avoid going to the garden center for anything because I feel like one of the kids who saw Willy Wonka's candy garden for the first time.

In order to properly outfit your little growing space, though, you do need a few supplies, and these come in handy:

- **Automatic light timers.** If you don't want to worry about turning lights on and off during a specific timeframe, these timers are very useful, and they're often fairly inexpensive. I use them when I'm going away for a weekend, or if I'll be busy for a stretch of time and want to reduce my indoor garden maintenance.

- **Heat mats.** Also called germination mats, these are designed to be placed underneath plants so that roots stay warm in cooler areas like basements or drafty corners. They're usually rectangular, and don't have temperature settings; you just roll them out, plug them in, put your pots or trays on top and you're good to go. The low temperature won't burn your plants (unlike, say, a heating pad would) and they do help during the winter months, I've found. Also, if your plants seem slow to germinate, using one of these can provide a boost. One caveat: they're usually not cheap, so if you see one on sale, snap it up.

- **Plastic mister bottle.** These are extremely useful, and only cost a few dollars. They can be utilized for an array of growing-related tasks, like spritzing fish emulsion on tomatoes, or spraying a soapy solution on aphid-ravaged plants. During certain times of year, my growing space feels a little drier than other times, so I often mist water over all the plants at least once per day.

- **Small plastic bins/totes.** Usually, I can get these for just a few bucks from places like Target, Family Dollar, or IKEA. Whenever there's a sale, I must look like a professional organizer, because I load up on them, especially ones that are about the size of a shoebox. Put everything in these that you need: scissors, twine, Sharpies, pens, light timers, rubber bands, etc. Also, these bins will be handy for organizing seeds; I tend to use several containers so I can sort seeds according to usage (pea shoot seeds in one bin, microgreens seed in another, and so on). I really wish that the rest of my house was as organized as my indoor gardening space.

Beyond the Backyard

When harvesting non-cultivated herbs—also known as wildcrafting or foraging—it's likely that your adventurous spirit might take you outside of your backyard, and into forests, prairies, parks, and other habitats. I applaud any sense of exploration, but please keep sustainability and safety in mind when you're doing any foraging. Some herbs become so popular that they get very overpicked, and then become endangered, or enthusiasts uproot the plant while harvesting, leaving whole patches of herbs unable to survive. And—know what you are picking!

Responsible foragers take only the flowers, leaves, or fruit that they're going to use, and leave the majority of the plant undisturbed. If you want to replant what you're taking in your own garden, try to take only the smallest amount of rootstock needed, or use seeds from the plant to place into the empty hole left behind. In general, though, foraging in a way that lets the area seem undisturbed is the best, and most responsible, way to harvest wild herbs.

Adventure: Round One

Whether you're noticing "weeds" that will prove useful, putting a few beloved herbs into a kitchen garden container, or creating an extensive medicinal herb garden that would make a Medieval monk blanch with envy, just enjoy the trip.

My herb garden is a work in progress, and it always will be, because every day, I'm learning about garden geek issues like soil health, fertilization, harvest dates, and pest control—but I'm also learning about patience, nourishment, awareness, and joy. When you look down into a cup of tea made from herbs that you planted, grew, harvested, and dried, there's a soul-quenching satisfaction that feels healing, before you even take a single sip.

Although I often embark on ambitious growing plans and find myself humbled time after time, I also appreciate that plants are a quiet and beautiful adventure, and I try to adjust my thinking accordingly. So, good luck on all your backyard pharmacy endeavors, and I'll raise a lemon-balm-infused cocktail to you, fellow traveler.

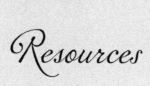

Resources

This guide to growing and using backyard medicinals is meant to be a starting point for any new gardening effort, especially for those who haven't tried growing any medicinal plants before. There are tons of wonderful resources out there that can expand your expertise and provide a wealth of indepth information. Here are some of my favorite resources.

BACKYARD BERRY PLANTS

www.backyardberryplants.com
This company specializes in organically grown blueberry, blackberry, and raspberry plants. In addition to being a supplier, the company has a wealth of information online about site preparation, plant care, and supplies. Be sure to check out the "other plants" section of the site for limited-time offers.

COOL SPRINGS PRESS

www.coolspringspress.com
In the spirit of full transparency, the book you're holding right now was published by Cool Springs Press, so maybe I'm a bit biased. But the publisher has tons of other great titles, so I consider my bias justified.

HIGH MOWING SEEDS

www.highmowingseeds.com
If you're looking for non-GMO, all-organic seeds, this is a great resource. They have a wide range of vegetables and herbs, as well as a blog about growing practices, food preservation, and other topics.

HORIZON HERBS

www.horizonherbs.com
One of the best-known seed companies in the world for medicinals, Horizon offers a huge array of herbs and other plants. They also feature mixes that are fun and economical, like the "Tasty Tea Collection" that puts together chamomile, fennel, hibiscus, spearmint, and tulsi, all for a price that's much lower than buying all those seed packets individually.

JOHNNY'S SELECTED SEEDS

www.johnnyseeds.com
This company is a treasured resource among farmers and gardeners, and for good reason. The site has videos, planting guides, herb growing charts, seed charts, and interactive tools.

JOURNAL OF HERBS, SPICES & MEDICINAL PLANTS

www.tandfonline.com/toc/whsm20/current

As you've probably noticed from the extensive use of academic studies included in this book, I love to geek out on research. There are many great journals that let me get my fix, and this is one of the best for glancing through. Many of the articles require a subscription, but you can view the abstracts for free.

MOUNTAIN ROSE HERBS

www.mountainroseherb.com

This is simply one of the best places ever to get herbal preparation supplies, from beeswax and carrier oils to multiple types of butters that are perfect for your medicinal concoctions. The company also hosts a series of free lectures by world-renowned herbalists that can be accessed online at freeherbalismproject.com.

PEACEFUL VALLEY

www.groworganic.com

This site is like catnip (or like catnip tea if that's your groove) for gardeners. Not only does it feature seeds, bare root trees, and plants, but you can also order greenhouses, frost protection, tools, and equipment.

SEED SAVERS EXCHANGE

www.seedsavers.org

This nonprofit organization is focused on saving and sharing heirloom seeds. Reading through the catalog is always compelling because they share little stories about where the seeds originated. They also provide very clear instructions about planting and tips for better growing.

SEEDS OF CHANGE

www.seedsofchange.com

Another strong choice for organic seeds, this site also has a nice collection of tools and supplies, including wooden planter boxes and "yield pots," which are lightweight, durable, and breathable options for an outdoor or indoor garden.

Index

chronic fatigue, 109
chronic pain, 55, 67
chronic stress, 146
cilantro, 14, 58–61
cleavers, 158
clover, red, 164
cold sores, 79
cold symptoms, 47, 54, 108, 109, 113, 120, 129, 142, 143. *See also individual symptoms*
colic, 63
colitis, 139
comfrey, 42, 43, 104–107
compost, 16
compresses, 40
concentration, 117, 125
constipation, 143, 160, 165
containers, 19, 20
coriander, 58–61
Coriandrum sativum, 58–61
coronary heart disease, 101
coughs, 63, 71, 83, 108, 109, 121, 139, 147, 160, 164
cramp bark, 34
culinary preparations, 37, 39

damiana, 43
dandelion, 37, 156, 159
dandruff, 75
decoctions, 39
dementia, 135
depression, 74, 78, 125, 135, 146, 159
dermatitis, 93, 147, 165
diabetes/blood sugar, 51, 59, 71, 75, 79, 135
diaper rash, 93
diarrhea, 135
digestion, 51, 55, 62, 63, 66, 67, 75, 78, 79, 97, 100, 117, 135, 143, 158, 161, 165
dill, 14
diuretics, 46, 139, 142, 156, 158

dry scalp, 75
drying plants, 37
dysentery, 139

ear infections, 120
earaches, 113, 121
echinacea, 108–111
Echinacea purpurea, 108–111
eczema, 147
elderberry, 27, 142–145
elemental sulfur, 17
energy boosters, 67
essential oil creations, 39
evening primrose, 125, 146–149
eye health, 135

fatigue, chronic, 109
fennel, 62–65
fertilizer, 16, 20, 27
feverfew, 47
fevers, 47, 129
fish emulsion, 16
flowers, 34
flu, 113, 142, 143
Foeniculum vulgare, 62–65
foraging, 167

garlic, 112–115
gas, 79
gastrointestinal wellness, 129, 147, 151
gingivitis. *See gum disease*
gingko, 43
gout, 135
ground ivy, 160
growing conditions, 14
growing supplies, 166
growth, maintaining, 27

Photo credits

Cool Springs Press: pp. 18

Tom Eltzroth: pp. 46 (top), 52, 116 (top), 122, 124 (top), 134 (top), 138 (top), 142 (top), 149

Katie Elzer-Peters: pp. 16 (right), 17 (right), 28 (all), 29 (all)

iStock: pp. 11, 88 (bottom)

Crystal Liepa: pp. 30

Elizabeth Millard: pp. 4, 8, 10 (both), 12, 15, 16 (left), 17 (left), 21, 24, 25, 26, 32, 34 (both), 35, 36, 37, 38 (all), 40, 41 (all), 42, 46 (bottom), 48, 49, 50 (bottom), 53, 54 (bottom), 58 (top), 62 (both), 64, 65, 66 (bottom), 68 (right), 70 (bottom), 72, 73, 74 (bottom), 76 (bottom), 80 (both), 82 (bottom), 84, 85, 86, 92 (bottom), 94, 100 (bottom), 103, 104 (bottom), 106, 107, 108 (bottom), 112 (bottom), 114 (both), 116 (bottom), 118, 120 (both), 124 (bottom), 126 (both), 128 (bottom), 130, 131, 146 (bottom), 156, 159, 161, 162, 163, 164

Jerry Pavia: pp. 146 (top)

Shutterstock: pp. 19, 44, 50 (top), 54 (top), 56, 57, 58 (bottom), 60, 61, 66 (top), 68 (left), 70 (top), 74 (top), 77, 78 (both), 82 (top), 88 (top), 90, 91, 92 (top), 95, 96 (both), 98, 99, 100 (top), 102, 104, (top), 108 (top), 110, 111, 112 (top), 119, 123, 128 (top), 132, 134 (bottom), 136, 137, 138 (bottom), 140, 141, 142 (bottom), 144 (both), 148, 150 (both), 152, 153, 154, 157, 158, 160, 165

Meet Elizabeth Millard

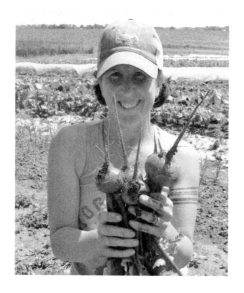

Elizabeth Millard and her partner Karla Pankow own Minnesota-based Bossy Acres, a farm that provides seasonal produce to community-supported agriculture members and area restaurants in an effort to build a strong and sustainable local food system. Millard often leads workshops on vegetable and herb gardening as well as herb preparation, fermentation, and cooking with seasonal ingredients. As a healthcare and wellness journalist and editor, she encourages readers to connect with the state's abundance of organic growers, ranchers, food artisans, nonprofit agencies, and one another, to forge a stronger food landscape.

In addition to farming, teaching, and editing, she has contributed articles to *Hobby Farm Home, Experience Life,* and *Urban Farm* magazines, along with many other publications. She and Karla share their home with their two impossibly spoiled dogs, Idgy and Ruthie Mae.

In addition to this book for Cool Springs Press, Elizabeth is the author of *Indoor Kitchen Gardening,* which focuses on practical tips for growing herbs, vegetables, and fruits in indoor settings. You can find Elizabeth in the garden, on Twitter @BossyEats, or on www.Facebook.com/BossyAcres (and also check out Karla @BossyAcres). Follow their adventures, and tell them about your own—they'd love to hear from you.

CPSIA information can be obtained
at www.ICGtesting.com
Printed in the USA
LVOW06s1931280817

546683LV00005B/5/P